THE WAY I SEE IT

A HEAD-TO-TOE GUIDE TO COMMON ORTHOPAEDIC CONDITIONS

To Bob: Enjoy! Regards,

Thomas

Thomas J. Neviaser, MD

First Edition copyright © 2015 Thomas J. Neviaser, MD

All rights reserved. No part of this publication may be reproduced, stored in a retrieval system, or transmitted in any form or by any means, electronic, mechanical, photocopying, recording, or otherwise, without the prior written permission of the publisher.

ISBN: 978-0-9760185-1-3

Printed in the United States of America

CONTENTS

Acknowledgements 7

Introduction 9

Chapter 1   The Office 13

Chapter 2   Occipital Nerve Headaches. 20

Chapter 3   The Neck (Cervical Spine) 24

Chapter 4   The Shoulder. 40

Chapter 5   The Collarbone (Clavicle) 76

Chapter 6   Upper Arm Bone (Humerus) 80

Chapter 7   The Elbow 82

Chapter 8   The Wrist. 91

Chapter 9   The Hand. 99

Chapter 10   The Thoracic Spine. 106

Chapter 11   The Thoracolumbar Spine. 112

Chapter 12   Lumbo-Sacral Spine. 114

Chapter 13	The Pelvis and Hip Joints	128
Chapter 14	The Knee	148
Chapter 15	The Tibia	185
Chapter 16	The Ankle	193
Chapter 17	The Foot	208
Chapter 18	Stress Fractures	225
Chapter 19	Osteoporosis	231
Chapter 20	Fibromyalgia	236
Chapter 21	Bone Healing	240
Chapter 22	The Operation	244
Chapter 23	Studies and Tests	254
Afterword		262
Glossary		263
Bibliography		271

DEDICATION

To all my patients who had the faith in me
as their physician and surgeon over the years,
and especially to my wife, Lynn, and my family
for their support despite my being absent
for many hours and days at a time.
I truly appreciate everything
all of you have done for me.

ACKNOWLEDGEMENTS

I must give credit to my former receptionists who remained with me for years, those whose personalities were perfect for dealing with all sorts of patients' feelings, and those who just got it right and understood the inherent problems of a medical practice and never let it get the best of them. I want to publicly thank all of them for their kindness and time spent helping me treat patients, especially Karen and Leslie. I must also thank those who helped in scheduling surgeries, a most difficult job to coordinate. Scheduling an operation with the hospital and the insurance companies is an arduous task in itself, but it takes even more time to deal with the patient's wants and fears in the laid-back manner that makes everything go as smoothly as possible. This is a skill few have, and when you find them, it's such a pleasure. If they don't have it, its lack can produce a great deal of friction that interferes with the final results. I was fortunate to have superb schedulers, especially Karen, Tanya, Trish, and Christie.

There's one more position I must talk about. Instead of dictating my histories and physical examinations, either after seeing the patient or at the end of the day, I always had a woman take notes for me while I interviewed the patient. The reason was twofold. I wanted a woman to be in the examining room for all female patients, and I had developed a modified shorthand and symbols that several people in the office could understand and from which quickly type a readable written history and exam. My employees called it Neviaser-eeze. Initially, Karen was the only one who could do it, but with time, others learned. As you can see, Karen was a help to me in many ways. When she was doing other things and/or retired, Mollie became her replacement and filled in admirably for many years. Later, she also helped in writing letters, typing drafts, and editing medical articles for publication. Often, she spent extra time helping me organize my presentations and papers for peer review journals as well. I want them all to know that I still appreciate every minute of their help because I certainly would have never accomplished what I did without them.

While I'm spreading of adulations, I would be remiss in not recognizing two of my longtime physical therapists who were often the main reasons I was able to have the great results I had—Barbara and Lilly. Believe me, just performing the surgery doesn't make it all work. Difficult times in therapy happen, and if you have dedicated, informed, sweet, and understanding people who have the skill, desire, and fortitude to stick with you in the tough times, your results will be above average. Both these ladies spent extra time and effort learning the anatomy and visiting the operating room to see what I did so they could incorporate that information into the postoperative therapy I prescribed. That type of dedication is difficult to find. They were truly troopers of extraordinary ability.

Thank you all, from the bottom of my heart.

INTRODUCTION

My wife and friends have asked me time and again to write something about my experiences in the practice of orthopedic surgery, but until now, I could never write anything I truly felt was worth a reader's time. Sure, there were some humorous and isolated instances that would be fun to write about, but I couldn't imagine anyone being interested in them.

With this book, I believe I have been successful in writing something instructive and worth people's time and effort to read and to help the reader understand what goes on inside their bodies.

Let's face it: medicine is a confusing, complicated, and often a totally misunderstood field of science. Physicians often believe they're in charge, and patients may conclude they have no choice other than trusting or not trusting their doctors. We doctors, on the other hand, are often too pressed for time to explain the causes of patients' symptoms in full, leaving so many of you feeling left out in the cold, not a participant in your own treatment.

After you visit a doctor, do you have a better sense of what's going on inside your body? Has she or he explained what parts of your body are involved, how they work together, or what's not working as it should so that you better understand your condition?

Being retired after practicing for more than thirty-five years, I'd like to share my orthopaedic experiences with you. I'm one of the three sons of an orthopaedic surgeon, and all of us became orthopaedic surgeons—a truly remarkable legacy. Whether our father knew it or not, even long after his death in 1980, he would continue to influence many lives for the better through his sons. While my brothers and I chose different medical schools and training programs, none of us would have traded our medical careers for anything else.

On the other hand, in preparation for our specialty and in the practice of it, we all had those few times when we asked ourselves, "What the heck were you thinking?" Over the years, most who sought my help for their bone and joint problems were pleasant, and I usually knew fairly soon what to do to help them. Then there were others who were the most diagnostically challenging cases I've ever treated and still others who were so obstinate, obnoxious, or making so much of their minuscule symptoms that they almost drove me crazy. Taken together, every one of them taught me something, helping me refine my approach to diagnosing and treating orthopaedic afflictions.

My purpose in writing this book is to publish an easy-to-read and understandable format that would help anyone with a personal interest in the subject—not medical professionals—just folks with a need to know why they hurt and what might be done to help. What I've laid out here is the way I see it; hence, the name of the book. While other orthopaedists may differ with my ideas, I found a logical approach to the diagnosis and treatment of orthopaedic disease processes that served me very well through the years, and I want to share them with you.

By the way, you may have noted my spelling of the word ORTHOPAEDIC. This is not a typographical error. My spell-check program busily scribbled a red line under this word every time I typed it, but what I've written is correct. "Orthopedic," the form more often seen today, is equally acceptable. However, because age has its privileges, and I'm a senior citizen, I prefer to follow the older version.

Once you've finished reading this book, I hope you'll have a good fundamental understanding, albeit from one clinical orthopaedist's view, of what happens when a certain symptom or combination of symptoms appears. I hope my attempts at simplifying complex explanations make sense to you. Not all of you may agree with me, and that's okay. At least you will have a basic starting point.

You have my promise to do my best to explain those big medical terms doctors use among themselves and, unfortunately, too often with their patients. One of my pet peeves has always been physicians bombarding patients with medical terms and never explaining what they mean. After seeking a doctor's help, I think it's far more important that the patients understand their bodily processes—the basis of their symptoms—than to memorize the medical labels applied to their problems. I would much rather that you grasp the big picture of your specific problem.

Because very complex processes underlie some of these conditions, you might find my attempts at scientific explanation confusing. I hope that won't happen, and I believe that if any of these common orthopaedic conditions should affect your way of life, this book will give you a better sense of what's going on in your body and why.

For organizational purposes, I've chosen to start from the head and end with the toes—a "head-to-toe guide to common orthopaedic conditions." One major category of orthopaedics you'll not find here is fractures: broken bones. There are just too many types of fractures to enumerate and explain, and the accepted treatments are too numerous, varied, and subject to change.

CHAPTER 1
THE OFFICE

I would like to begin by talking about what occurs daily in an orthopaedist's office. Having had my own busy office practice as well as having visited other doctors' offices for myself and with my wife, my children, and my grandchildren, I know how frustrating it is to sit for what seems an unnecessarily long time in a doctor's waiting room and in the examining room as well once you've made it that far.

Over coffee or at the water cooler at work, folks always discuss how long they had to wait to get in to see a doctor. Why was he so late? Why did they schedule me so close to others? What could he be doing that's so important? Understandable questions, but they really do have logical answers.

First, every physician's office has one or more persons known as "schedulers" who make up the daily schedule. That person schedules appointments for folks wanting to be seen, and in a surgeon's practice, the same person may also schedule operations. Practices with a heavy surgical load or multiple doctors may have a second scheduler just for operations. The schedules for office visits and operations must be coordinated, and sometimes, many last-minute changes are necessary.

Patients calling to make an appointment are divided into two major groups: new patients and established ("old") patients. The new patients fall into two groups:

- Folks with just one complaint.
- Folks with more than one problem.

Established patients fall into three groups:
- Those with a new problem.
- Those in for follow-up on an old complaint.
- Those in for a postoperative checkup.

The scheduler is expected to reserve an appropriate amount of time for each patient to be seen. A scheduler who's been with the doctor for a long time may be expert at it, but those in an office with a high staff turnover may not be so skillful. Believe me, it is a very demanding job, and a great deal of skill and practice is needed to become proficient. Placing a novice in this position is a disaster about to happen.

Why not just draw up an all-purpose schedule with appropriate time slots for the various groups? More time for a new patient, less for established patients unless they have new problems, and still less for postoperative visits—shouldn't that work? On paper it is plausible, but in reality, all kinds of problems throw that type of schedule off. For instance, suppose Mrs. Brown comes in for evaluation of her painful knee. If she and Dr. Ortho use the entire fifteen-minute appointment getting to the nitty-gritty of her problem, fine. But once she's in the doctor's presence, if Mrs. Brown proceeds to tell him her shoulder also bothers her or asks advice about her husband's bad back or her daughter's tennis elbow—in short, taking up more of Dr. O's time than was allotted for her—the schedule is already out of whack for the rest of the day.

If Dr. O's polite, doing his best to hear all Mrs. Brown's concerns, he's taking away from the time he needs to ask questions to help him diagnose her main problem. And unless she answers his questions and sticks to the point, more time is lost.

All the while, in the waiting room Mr. Jones, Ms. Green, and little Tommy Fidget and his mother sit, wondering why they aren't being seen on time. If this happens repeatedly with twenty-five or thirty folks, by day's end, Dr. Ortho will be two hours behind, and the whole waiting room will be unhappy, if not irate.

Mrs. Brown or Mr. Jones may not like it if the doctor, needing to get his questions back on track, interrupts their digressions from their original complaints. They may think their concerns haven't received appropriate attention. I'm not talking about the doctor who just doesn't plainly listen or gives you his full attention. I know that type of unprofessional behavior is a huge turnoff. But if you, Mr. Jones, or Mrs. Brown will help the doctor stick to the subject and keep to the schedule, then the folks in the waiting room will be seen at or close to their scheduled time, and everyone will be very grateful for it.

But then the unexpected happens!

It's 3:00 p.m. The doctor's office gets a call from the high school practice field, reporting that Peyton Favre, the star quarterback, has been sent to the emergency room with a bad knee injury. He's in a lot of pain. He can't bear weight on it, and Dr. O.'s on call. Peyton's dad wants him to be seen right away. Dr. O. instructs the ER physician to send the boy to his office for an examination to rule out any hidden emergency and plan the treatment. This time-consuming incident can easily disturb the office schedule.

Or suppose the nursing home calls to say Mrs. A tried to get out of bed without assistance, fell in the bathroom, and has apparently broken her hip. What should Dr. O do? He has to spend time evaluating the emergency condition of the patient over the phone and then set in motion a plan for immediate treatment and possible emergency surgery for her.

Or the emergency room calls to tell Dr. O. that his wife's nephew has been involved in an automobile accident, shattering his ankle, and won't have anybody but Dr. O. Dr. O has to get through his appointments quickly so he can go to the hospital to see about the boy.

I think you're getting the idea. Incidents like this happen every day. Time must be made for these folks too. Some offices schedule emergency time slots, but the emergencies don't always wait for those scheduled times. And some days are just plain crazy, with more folks than usual showing up in the waiting room.

It's not the easiest job in the world, checking all the folks who need to be seen and keeping the schedule running like clockwork. One of my patients complained constantly about the time "wasted" in my office. "I should charge you for my time," she often jested. Finally, I offered her the job of scheduler! I told her I would start her at $50,000 a year plus a healthy bonus, if she could schedule my days so that no patients complained about having to wait. She never took me up on my offer, but she did stay with me as a patient, so I guess she just had to let off some steam. I understood her frustrations, though. Doctors and their staff just can't anticipate every snafu. I wish I could have, and if any of you have the answer, I hope you'll let me know!

Sometimes, a schedule gone awry is entirely the doctor's fault. He may spend too much time on hospital rounds, lose track of time, and show up late at the office. He might spend too much time on the telephone during office hours. I always answered other doctors but told the callers that I was seeing patients and, if need be, would call back at the end of the day. Many times, I didn't have to call back as they usually knew the situation and were ready to tell me their problems quickly, and I had an easy time dealing with them. A more complex case would certainly be a scheduling nightmare.

A young doctor, hoping to impress a patient with his intense interest, may take too long seeing him. The person getting the attention will be impressed, but the physician probably soured others who had to wait.

Talking about things other than medicine will definitely damage the scheduled time. Office hours aren't the time for social chitchat. I confess I've been guilty of it, but I tried to resist the temptation. Doctors are only human, just like the folks who come to us for care.

And some botched schedules are partly the doctor's fault as well as the patients'. Frustration builds in the waiting room, and especially at the receptionist's desk. The staff gets antsy because patients' frustration and discontent are contagious. The receptionist on the front line catches the heat, but it usually is not her fault. Bad feelings can persist, even after folks go home, setting up distrust between them and the doctor.

I just have to tell you about an unusual incident that absolutely destroyed my office schedule one day. I was interrupted by my secretary that one of my partner's patient was on the phone, believe it or not, canceling his appointment since he was about to commit suicide. Honestly, I kid you not. I was on the phone with this man for three hours, attempting to talk him out of it while writing notes to my secretary to call the police and have the call traced. Tracing a call evidently is not as easy as it seems on television. Finally, I was notified that the police were on their way and was to keep close contact with him. In the end, they found him, and a death was averted. One of the policemen asked if I wanted him brought to the office, and I politely replied, "I'm an orthopaedist, not a psychiatrist. Please take him to the nearest hospital for care." I had sixteen patients in the waiting room and sitting on the floor in front of me while I corresponded with this man. They all applauded the successful ending. Office hours ran into the night that day.

There is an epilogue to this story. Three to four weeks later, I was interrupted by my secretary, telling me I had an important phone call. It was this man calling to thank me for saving his life. Sometimes, life can be beautiful in the midst of all its confusion.

If and when you do see the doctor, here are a few suggestions that may help make the best use of your appointment time.

1. Before you go, write down your complaint as you want to explain it to the doctor.
2. Make notes about the questions that follow to keep you on track at the visit.
3. If you have several problems, describe the most severe one first, then the others, in as few words as you can.
4. Be ready for questions about the location of the pain, when it started, whether it followed an injury, whether you have had the same pain before, and so on.
5. Be ready to give a concise history without going off on a tangent.
6. Describe treatments another doctor has prescribed or those you have tried.
7. Carry your notes with you when you go!
8. Before your appointment, if another doctor referred you, call that doctor and arrange to pick up your medical records, X-rays, and reports of any studies to bring with you. If the referring doctor offers to send the material, check ahead of time to be sure it was done.
9. If you're always fearful about seeing a doctor (the white coat syndrome), arrange to bring your spouse, another family member, or a friend along.
10. If you're nervous, tell the doctor and ask him to repeat the diagnosis and proposed treatment for you. If necessary, ask him to write it down. Don't let the big medical words go by without asking what they mean or asking to have them explained.

11. If you don't understand, say so. Don't just nod yes in hopes of getting out as soon as possible.

12. Always review the proposed treatment with the doctor to be sure you understand and can follow the instructions. If you think you might not be able to follow them, tell the doctor so.

13. If you sense that the doctor is not completely focused on your problem, offer to come back at a more convenient time. Nine times out of ten, this will jolt him and redirect his attention.

14. Above all, realize you're not the only person being seen that day.

15. Respect the doctor's and the other patients' time.

So you see, a doctor's office schedule is more complicated than you might have imagined. Inevitably, some folks will have to wait—a short time at best but sometimes longer. Those unavoidable delays will frustrate you as they also frustrate the doctor. Ideally, we all want to keep to a predictable schedule, but realistically, it simply doesn't always happen in spite of our best efforts.

CHAPTER 2
OCCIPITAL NERVE HEADACHES

Headaches? Why start an orthopaedic guide with headaches? If you suffer from headaches at the back of your head or the top of your neck that your physician has investigated fully without identifying the cause, you may be referred to an orthopaedic surgeon.

Right now is a good time to point out that we human beings are home to a vast and very complicated network of nerves, branching out from the spinal cord to all parts of our bodies, and when something is amiss with one of these nerves, we may feel pain. Doctors refer to a particular nerve by name depending on what part of the body it serves. In this case, the affected nerve serves the lower back of the head, the *occiput* [OX-sa-put], so we describe pain as *occipital* [ox-SIP-pit-tal] in nature, hence the diagnosis of *occipital headaches*.

Located at the base of the back of the head, on either the right or the left, these headaches occur when compression or irritation affects the *greater occipital nerve*, which emerges from the base of the skull off-center, one on the right and one on the left (Fig. 1). This nerve runs toward the middle of the base of your skull, then quickly turns ninety degrees upward through some small muscles to become *subcutaneous* [sub-kew-TAIN-e-us], meaning "under the skin," and gives sensation to the skin in this area.

With age, inflammation, or just plain irritation over time, the nerve can produce pain that folks describe as a headache.

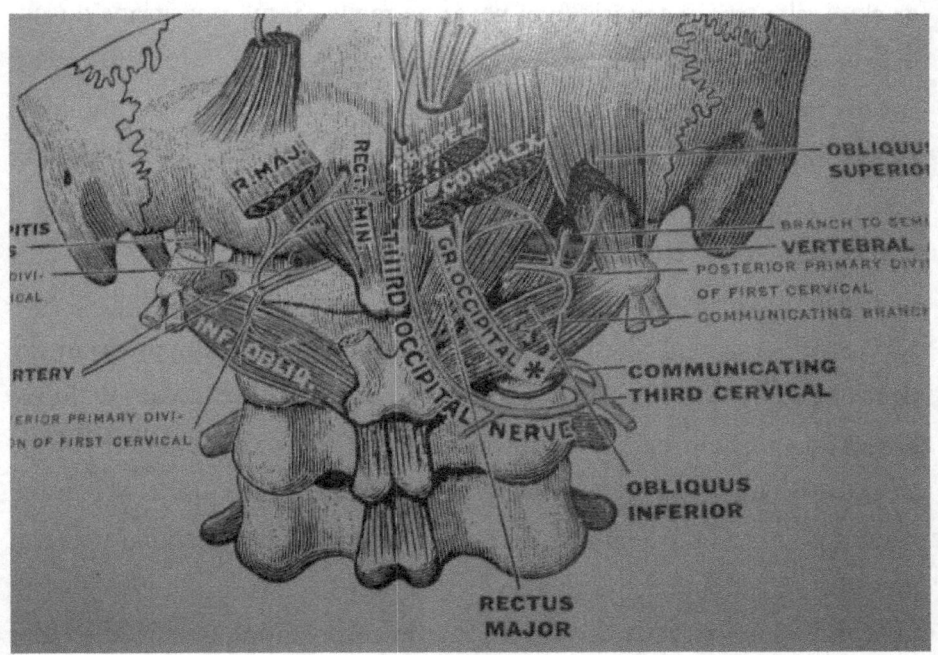

Fig. 1: The base of the skull and upper spine.
The right greater occipital nerve (* wide structure); note its acute turn upward as it exits the skull.
Gray's Anatomy, 1966

What can be done to relieve these headaches? Various treatments have been tried, alone or in combination, including anti-inflammatory medication, wet heat, physical therapy, massage, ultrasound and electrical stimulation, acupuncture, holistic therapy, and chiropractic manipulation, with varying degrees of success. Your doctor will probably prescribe some or all of these same treatments for other conditions we discuss because for many orthopaedic conditions, these therapies are the first line of treatment; therefore, I'll probably refer to many of these treatments often throughout this book.

Because folks who suffer from occipital headaches or doctors who see those folks may believe they're dealing with actual "aches" inside the head or skull, the true diagnosis may never be made. Some physicians do not believe in this specific diagnosis. I'm not certain why. For initial treatment, the doctor may try a "shotgun" approach in the hope that even though a diagnosis hasn't been fully made, time and one of these treatments will take care of the problem. I say this with confidence because, I regret to say, I have also used this technique in the past.

I believe that if the doctor will take time to ask for a thorough history and carry out careful physical examination, he can generally pinpoint the painful area. A single instruction, "Point to the area of your pain with one finger," may be all that's needed. If the doctor knows the anatomy of the area, the occipital nerve can usually be identified as the culprit. When the patient points to the anatomical location of the greater occipital nerve, it may well be the source of the pain.

In my practice, when a person came in complaining of this off-center headache and pointed to this area, I often found a pinpoint tenderness there. Other types of headaches (migraines, for example) usually will not exhibit pinpoint areas of tenderness. Injecting this "trigger point"—an area of greatest tenderness—with a short-acting local anesthetic such as Lidocaine may cause the pain to vanish for a short period of time, thereby proving that this specific area is the cause of the symptoms. Adding a refined steroid to this injection may reduce the inflammation or irritation of the nerve even longer.

Injecting this trigger point on the first visit can eliminate the need for other treatments, saving time and money and bringing immediate relief rather than allowing the pain to continue while other treatments are scheduled, waited for, and undergone without success, only to have the patient come back weeks or months later with the same symptoms. Long-term treatment may necessitate occasional injections followed by physical therapy; however, the injection usually did the trick in my hands most of the time.

The goal of a doctor should be to make the earliest possible diagnosis, followed by the most advantageous and effective treatment. Sending the patient off for six weeks of therapy without a true diagnosis never made much sense to me. Eliminating the pain on the first office also gives the patient great relief, the doctor a feeling of accomplishment, and a mutually beneficial doctor-patient relationship is established quickly even though the symptoms may return later.

Posterior Auricular Neuritis

This another neuritis is similar to the occipital neuritis we just discussed. *Auricular* [aw-RICK-cue-lar] refers to the ear, and *posterior* means "behind"; therefore, the affectation is an inflammation of the posterior auricular nerve, which is located behind the ear at the base of the skull. I know this entity exists because I have had it and despite anti-inflammatory medications, including oral cortisone, my pain—severe at times—was not relieved until the trigger point of tenderness was injected with a refined steroid and local anesthetic. The local anesthetic permits the physician injecting the area a quick feedback as to whether he was in the correct area. As for me, I could tell my physician had hit it directly because the majority of my pain was relived within thirty to forty-five seconds. Over the next few days, the pain dissipated and disappeared totally.

CHAPTER 3
THE NECK (CERVICAL SPINE)

Cervical [SIR-vick-al] *spine* is the medical term for the uppermost portion of the spine. It is derived from the Latin word *cervix*, which means "neck." In this chapter, we'll talk about common neck problems that may cause you to be referred to an orthopaedic surgeon.

There is a very simple way to identify true neck pain for yourself. Should your neck hurt whenever you move your head from side to side, up or down, or during rotation, the problem probably lies within your neck itself. On the other hand, if moving your head in those directions doesn't make your neck hurt, it's time to look elsewhere for the cause.

One of my dearest friends called me from New York, telling me his cardiologist (a heart specialist) had sent him to an orthopaedic surgeon for his neck pain. He described his visit and said this orthopaedist had recommended a treatment similar to what I described in chapter 2 for occipital headache. When I asked him to move his head in all directions, he told me none of these motions brought on his neck pain. He was soon coming down for a visit, so I waited until I saw him to give my opinion about his condition.

The day after he arrived, he accepted my invitation to go duck hunting. During our half-mile walk to the duck blind, I noticed that with every thirty or forty yards, he would stop and rub his neck. Once we were in the blind, I asked him to move his head again to see if it brought on the pain. It did not.

At that point, I knew he had *referred pain*—pain felt in one part of the body but caused by a problem in another part. In his case, the real problem was his heart. He had *angina pectoris* [AN-jine-a PEC-tor-is], pain from a clog in one or more of the coronary arteries that supply blood to the heart muscle. His angina was not typical since he only felt the pain in his neck, whereas most folks complain of chest pain.

Even though his cardiologist had sent him to an orthopaedic specialist, I urged him to see a second cardiologist when he returned home. He did so, and within five days, he had undergone a quadruple coronary bypass. His neck pain disappeared. From this story, you can see that not all neck pain originates in the neck.

True neck pain is not usually felt just in the neck, however. Often, it's referred to the *trapezius* [tra-PEA-zee-us] muscles, the large muscles that spread from the base of the neck across the top of your shoulders (Fig. 2). In fact, pains here without neck pain may be the only symptom emanating from the cervical spine.

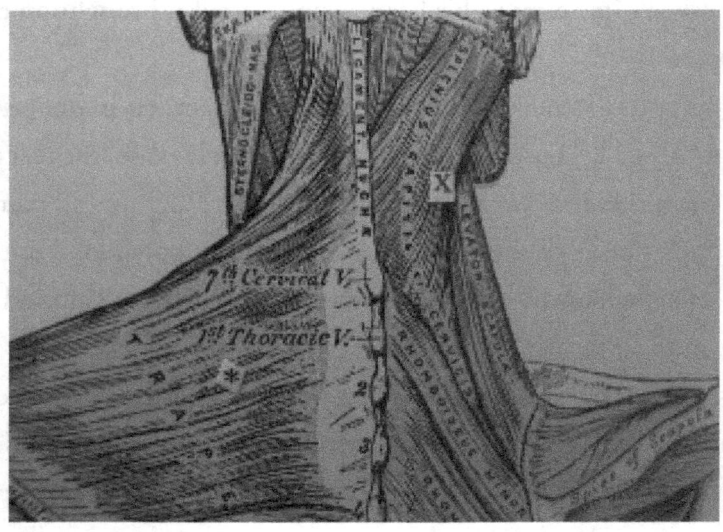

Fig. 2: Left: the trapezius muscle; (*) marks the area of neck "referred pain." Right: paravertebral muscles of the neck (x).
Gray's Anatomy, 1966

Many folks think of these muscles as their shoulders, but they aren't, and insisting their "shoulder" or "shoulders" are bothering them often convinces the examiner that they really mean their shoulder joints. I have seen this mistake made many times over. That is why the initial instruction should be, "Point to your area of pain with one finger." When they point to the trapezius muscle, the examiner will not be misled by their misnomer. Referred pain from the cervical spine may be described as a bee sting or deep pinpoint ache directly in the center of these trapezius muscles, and certain motions of the neck will increase this pain. Rubbing the painful area can give temporary relief, but it soon returns because the pain is coming from the neck, usually as a result of a fragmenting or degenerative *disc*.

Everyone has heard of a slipped disc, but what exactly does this mean? A disc does not really slip; it fragments within its space and loosens up. When this fragmented tissue pushes, bulges against, and stretches the ligaments that hold it in place, pain is almost always felt or "referred" to areas in the neck and the trapezius muscles. Many patients swear they can pinpoint the pain directly over the muscle because they can feel it "right there." They just know their symptoms are muscular in origin. There's a simple explanation for this. When someone rubs and massages the area for relief many times a day, or even for weeks at a time, this spot becomes quite sensitive. Simply pressing or touching it then produces a pain, but it's not really the same pain arising from the real culprit, a disc in the neck. This is a difficult premise to explain and have the patient understand. The patient will usually complain of pain over either the right or the left trapezius muscle, rarely both. Why? Let's look more closely at the makeup and anatomy of these discs.

If you've seen a skeleton, you know that the spine looks like a long chain of similar-looking bones. Each individual bone is called a *vertebra* [VER-ta-bra]; the plural is *vertebrae* [VER-ta-bray]. A vertebra has three parts: the large, round, canister-shaped part, which bears most of the weight, is known as the *centrum*; behind the centrum is the *vertebral* [ver-TEE-bral] *arch* or *dorsal arch*, which protects the spinal cord and the nerves within the circle created. It also has two (right and left) oblong outcroppings or processes covered by a white glistening surface, which make up one half of the joints (*facet joints*) that connect each vertebra to another. Finally, the pointed midline outgrowth of this arch is the *spinous process*, or spine of the vertebra (Fig. 3).

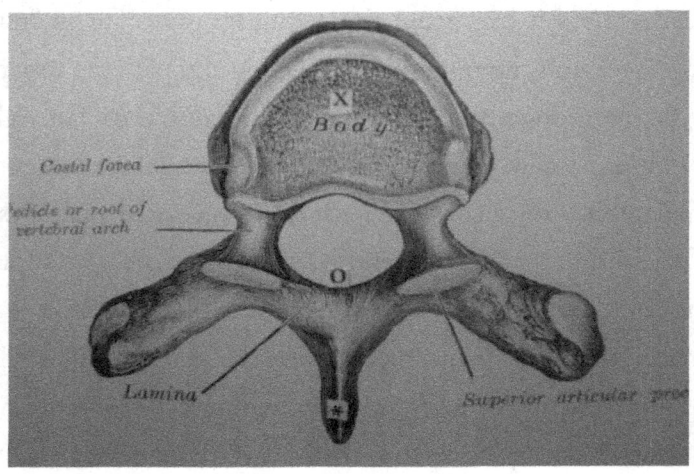

Fig. 3: A vertebra: X marks the centrum (body),
O marks the arch, and * marks the spinous process.
Note the two oblong joint processes that will articulate with the next
vertebra's processes to form facet joints
Gray's Anatomy, 1966

If you run your finger down the middle of someone's neck or back, you can usually feel the tips of these spinous processes, and if the person is quite thin, you can actually see the tips as well. Each vertebra is separated from the one above and below by an *intervertebral* [inter-ver-TEE-bral] *disc* and circumferential ligaments holding them all together.

A normal disc has a semi-gelatinous center, the *nucleus pulposus* [NEW-klee-us pul-PO-sus], surrounded by a dense ring of fibrous cartilage material called the *annulus fibrosis* [AN-ew-lus fie-BRO-sis)] (Fig. 4)—*annulus* meaning "ring" in Latin, and *fibrosis* meaning many fibers.

The Neck (Cervical Spine)

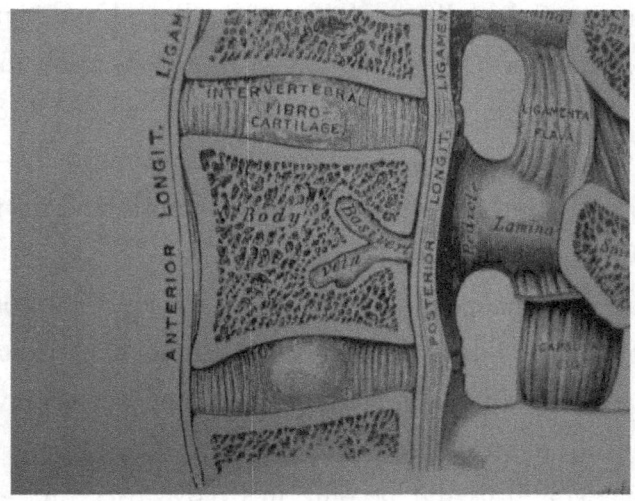

Fig. 4: The intervertebral disc: annulus fibrosis (fibrocartilage), top space, Nucleus pulposus, central oblong structure, lower space.
Gray's Anatomy, 1966

This intervertebral disc is formed in such a way that forces placed upon it are dissipated throughout the disc space by the central nucleus pulposus, allowing flexibility of the spine and equal distribution of forces. A simplified way to think of it is by comparing the disc to a golf ball—a really old one, not the kind made today.

As a child, any time I got hold of one with a crack in it, I would remove the white cover and unravel what seemed a mile of rubber-band material to find a little rubber sphere filled with a thick jellylike substance. This made a terrific super ball because this little sphere could be bounced high in the air and seemingly would keep bouncing almost forever. It certainly kept my attention for hours. I guess you can say this was my Xbox of the day.

The combination of rubber bands and super ball core carried any force from outside the golf ball to its center where it is reversed, sending the force back from whence it came. When a golfer teed off for a drive, the force of his striking the ball traveled to the bands and eventually to the jelly core, making the ball spring off the club head and fly forward. I believe the semi-gelatinous intervertebral disc, with its surrounding fibrous material, reacts to outside forces in a very similar way—a marvelous mechanical wonder. You could say, by compressing this type of golf ball down to a pancake shape, the white covering of a golf ball represents ligaments around the disc, the rubber bands represent the annulus fibrosis, and the super ball is the nucleus pulposus.

But what would happen to the golf ball if the super ball core dried up? The force of the club hitting the golf ball would not be distributed equally, right? The ball wouldn't go far, and hitting it time and again would cause the rubber bands to break under the stress.

These old golf balls did become ineffective over time because the center would dry up, and the rubber bands would eventually fragment and break. I believe something very much like this happens in our bodies, probably as early as age twenty. For some reason, the "super ball core" of our intervertebral discs dries up; water is absorbed from the gelatinous center. No one knows why, but this type of phenomenon occurs in many other areas of the body as you will see.

When it happens, the surrounding fibers—the *annulus fibrosis*—bear the brunt of forces placed on the spine in the course of a day. Doing a job they weren't designed for, these fibrous rings fragment over time, breaking into small pieces like chunks of crab meat. These fragments (Fig. 6) can't distribute the forces from outside, and those forces eventually get the upper hand, pushing the fragments around. In turn, the fragments press repeatedly against ligaments, and the ligaments give and stretch, bulging outward at the weakest point, usually on the right or the left of the back side or posterior aspect of the disc space (Fig. 5).

Like any bodily tissue that's stretched, such as gas-filled intestines or a fluid full urinary bladder, a stretched ligament causes pain that may be referred to nearby muscles. In the case of a bulging cervical disc, it's the trapezius muscles we discussed above.

As mentioned, many patients, and even some doctors, diagnose these referred pains as "muscle strains" or "muscle spasms," when the pain actually is emanating from the cervical spine by stretched intervertebral ligaments. A true muscle strain is rare. Hamstring muscles tear, and thigh muscles can be strained by overload, but short, stocky muscles like the trapezius, whose fibers have very little distance to travel, rarely become strained for no known reason.

As for spasms, a muscle doesn't spasm unless it has a reason. For example, night cramps, potassium deficiency, lactic acid overload, or the need to protect an area from further injury. Physical therapists often tell patients they can feel a muscle in spasm, generally on either side of the neck just under the trapezius muscle, so they try to relax these muscles through massage. In fact, therapists often massage the muscle directly over the first rib and, feeling the rib, may conclude that the muscle is in spasm.

When a cervical disc suddenly bulges, however, the *paravertebral* [para-ver-TEE-bral] muscles (Fig. 2) surrounding the cervical spine will spasm, causing decreased neck motion. This spasm is protective, limiting neck motion to protect and allowing time for the bulge to subside. This restriction of motion is the stiffness and inability to turn the neck.

To explain, let's go a step further. Old tires used to be made with an inner tube inside. When the side walls became weak, the inner tube would bulge at the weakest point, splitting the outside wall of the tire. Likewise, as the fragmented disc material increases pressure and bulges, it will eventually balloon through the weakest point (Fig. 6) and split the ligament. Result? More referred pain. When the disc bulges well beyond the disc space, it irritates a nerve traveling through this area, and this also can refer pain along that nerve down the arm. Someone with a bulging cervical disc may also have spells of numbness and tingling in the arm as a result of this phenomenon.

Although these episodes can last from three to six weeks, most of the time, the disc material either returns to the disc space or is gradually absorbed by the body. Pressure on the ligament is relieved, the bulging disappears, and, fortunately, the pain subsides. The first line of conservative treatments mentioned above, along with steroid medication given by mouth, often helps bring the episode to an end more quickly.

On the other hand, if the disc bulges so much that the ligament can no longer contain it, a disc fragment may ooze out of the disc space—a *herniated disc* (Fig. 6). This can happen quickly or slowly. If the herniated disc is large enough, it will press on the nearby nerve, causing constant numbness, tingling, and pain over the area the nerve supplies. The ligament—still stretched—continues to produce pain in the neck and those same big muscles, the trapezii.

If a piece of disc material completely vacates its space, no longer stretching the ligament, pain may actually disappear from the trapezius muscle and the neck so that the patient's only complaints are related to nerve compression: numbness, tingling, and pain in the arm. The space in which these discs herniate is so extremely small that there's no room for compromise in treatment. If short-term treatment doesn't relieve the symptoms, the only option may be surgery.

Let's take a look at these ligaments so you can get an idea of the whole picture. Ligaments connect one vertebra to the next and hold the discs in place. Along the central back part of a person's vertebrae, the ligaments are much larger and stronger, thinning out a bit toward the sides, then becoming thicker again, leaving a potentially weak area on the right and the left back sides of a disc space (Fig.5).

The Neck (Cervical Spine)

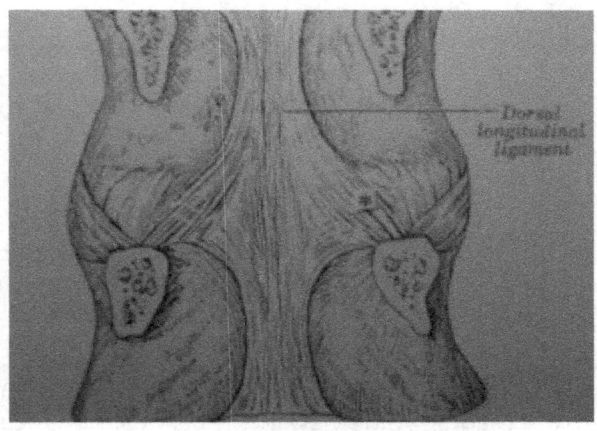

Fig. 5: Posterior spinal ligaments:
Note thinning areas of the posterior ligaments
on the right (*) and left
Gray's Anatomy 1966

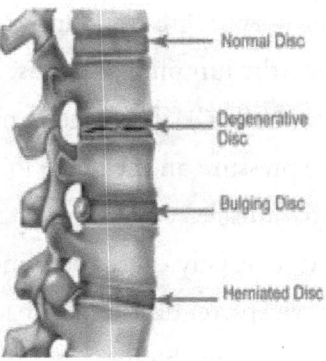

Fig. 6: Diagram of different disc conditions
Beverly Hills Pain Management Center Website

The cervical spine includes seven vertebrae (Fig. 7), identified as C1 through C7. The most common cervical disc herniations seen in my practice were at C5-6 and C6-7, with a few at C4-5.

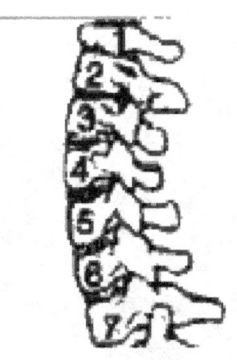

Fig. 7: Diagram: Side view of the cervical spine (C)
with numbered vertebrae
www.Sci-Info-Pages.com

Herniations of the disc at C5-6 will produce pain in the neck, over the trapezius muscle, over the upper the arm (with numbness and tingling), and, if compression of the nerve is great enough, a reduced or absent biceps tendon reflex at the elbow (the jumping of a muscle when your doctor taps its tendon is known as a "reflex"). The biceps muscle may also become quite weak because of the pressure on the nerve in the neck short circuiting the electrical signals to the muscle.

At C6-7, a herniated disc usually causes pain in the elbow and the lower arm, reduced or absent triceps tendon reflex (back upper portion of the elbow), numbness and tingling in the forearm and the hand, and possibly weakness of the triceps muscle.

If your doctor finds that you have *neurologic deficits* [new-row-LODGE-gick DEAF-uh-sits]—numbness, muscle weakness, or both, indicating pressure on a nerve—surgery must be considered because prolonged pressure on any nerve can cause permanent weakness and numbness. Sometimes, unfortunately, the nerve damage persists, even after pressure on that nerve is relieved.

What should you expect from surgery for a single herniated cervical disc causing neurologic changes? Results can range from quite good to excellent. The operation is usually performed from the front of the neck, where the discs can be more easily approached and removed. The entire disc is removed, and the surgeon can see the offending disc fragment compressing the nerve and remove it as well. To keep the nerve tunnels, the *neural foraminae* [new-ral for-AY-men-aye]—open and to avert any further irritation of the nerve—the surgeon will insert bone fragments (Fig.8) and possibly metallic plates to stabilize them and eventually fuse two vertebrae together. This bone fusion is known as *arthrodesis* [ar-throw-DEE-sis].

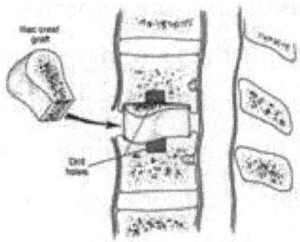

Fig. 8: Diagram of bone graft fragment replacing cervical disc.
www.spinalneurosurgery.com

In deciding whether to have the operation, you will be told that any surgery carries the possibility of complications. But even though no one looks forward to an operation on his neck, if a herniated disc causes enough pain and disturbance in your everyday life, surgery is definitely worth considering. Ask your surgeon to tell you several things:

- What procedure he plans
- Any possible complications
- What your limitations will be immediately afterward
- How long you will take to recover

You can then decide whether to go ahead although I always encouraged my patients to get a second opinion.

When stiffness of your neck gradually becomes apparent over a long period of time, the cause probably isn't pure disc disease itself but arthritic changes in the facet [FA-set] joints that are a part each vertebra and allow motion between it and the vertebrae above and below. Over the years, disc degeneration and deterioration without herniation will occur in all disc spaces, and the slow loss of height eventually can cause an offset of the joints behind them, leading to degenerative arthritis with referred pain. Referred where? You guessed it—the trapezius muscles. Treating this pain is a longer process, and while the pain may be substantially reduced, it can't always be eliminated. Surgery is not often indicated for this condition.

Remember then that not all neck pain is related to a diseased disc, and true neck pain can usually be reproduced by certain neck motions. There are certainly other obscure diagnoses for neck pain, but we're focusing here on the most common pain patterns and conditions seen in an orthopaedic surgeon's office.

"Whiplash" Injuries

Often used to refer to an acute sprain of the ligaments, strained muscles of the neck, or both, the term *whiplash* is really a misnomer. Many folks believe that in certain situations, especially automobile accidents, the force of the accident tosses the head forward and backward like a whip. I don't agree. When struck from behind, the body is driven forward while the head lags behind momentarily before catching up. Immediately, the neck muscles tense and contract to stop the head from moving too fast and too far forward. For that reason, I don't see this as a true whiplash motion. What happens then is that the involved muscles and ligaments are microscopically injured, strained, or sprained.

Simply put, muscle injuries are *strains*, and ligament injuries are *sprains*.

Even though the terms *sprain* and *strain* are often used interchangeably, I will refer to a ligament injury as a *sprain* and an injury to a muscle as a *strain*.

Regardless of what you call it, this type of injury causes pain although it may be delayed for several reasons. First, the victim's mental and physical reactions to the mishap may overcome any awareness of pain. More pressing problems may cause the person to ignore the neck pain for a short time. If the injury is mild to moderate, swelling and inflammation may become noticeable only after some time. Finally, some folks just have a high pain threshold and will not feel the results for a while. In any case, within a day or two, the injured person will definitely feel discomfort or pain, if the episode caused enough injury.

The appropriate treatment, either by the emergency room staff or at a doctor's office, includes medication for pain and to decrease inflammation as well as immobilization of the neck, usually by a soft collar. The use of the collar is limited to three to four weeks, but many folks continue wearing theirs for months. Healing begins very soon after the accident, and if the neck is immobilized for too long, the injured ligaments and muscles heal in a scarred and shortened form. After several weeks, when the collar is removed, the injured person may complain of limited neck motion with pain similar to the pain of the original injury.

At that point, mistakenly believing the injury hasn't healed, he or she will almost invariably put the collar back on—a big mistake. Time and again, I saw the results of this terrible cycle in folks who eventually came to me for a second opinion. I always told them to totally eliminate the collar right away and gave them specific exercises for stretching the healed, shortened ligaments and muscles. Rather than referring them to a physical therapist, I encouraged them to perform their own exercises and made it clear that while these would cause pain, they would not cause any harm. Then I closely monitored them, the length of time depending on the individual case. The longer they had worn the collar, the longer it would take to rehabilitate them after they took it off.

Whenever someone came to me with a new injury, I had them wear the collar for just five days or so and then started them on gradual but intense home exercises to stretch the ligaments and muscles as they healed. By the time these injured areas were restored, the person usually had regained a normal range of neck motion.

Someone with a neck injury sustained in an accident may consult an attorney to institute a lawsuit, and while I won't dwell on the subject of lawsuits generated by neck injuries, I have been called as an expert witness in cases where the pain occurred weeks after the accident. I don't believe a car accident could cause such delayed symptoms. On the other hand, attorneys tend to tie the extent of injury to the damage to the car or cars, but I contend that the body's normal reaction to this type of mechanical force is always an acute, full reflex contraction of the muscle, no matter how minor the accident.

Congenital Cervical Torticollis

A *congenital cervical torticollis* [con-JEN-it-al SUR-vick-al tor-ti-COLL-is] means an anatomic twisting and tilting of the neck from birth. Some have termed it *wry neck*. Usually noticed within two to four weeks of age, doctors attribute it to an injury sustained in the uterus or at birth that caused *fibrosis* (scarring) and *contracture* (shortening) of the *sternocleidomastoid* [ster-no-cly-do-MAS-toid] *muscle*—a long, thin, flat muscle that runs from the back of each ear down the side of the neck to the collarbone and the sternum.

Infants with this condition are often unable to fully rotate or bend the head to one side. Typically, the head tilts toward the affected muscle and is turned toward the opposite side. Early treatment is essential because unless the torticollis is corrected, the face can become misshapen. A child with torticollis should be followed closely by a doctor familiar with the condition to make sure the face doesn't become deformed.

The first form of treatment is stretching to correct the tightness, sometimes with a collar to prevent more contracture. If stretching fails to correct the problem, a few of these children will need surgery to release the muscle.

Congenital torticollis is not to be confused with *acquired torticollis*, a tilting of the head and neck caused by muscle spasms from any of a number of causes, including an acute herniated disc, as discussed above.

CHAPTER 4
THE SHOULDER

For many years, I specialized in conditions of the shoulder, one of the most complicated and versatile joints in the human body, allowing a variety of positions and uses of the arm and hand. The information in this chapter is what I have learned over the many years of dealing with patients and their shoulder problems.

Patients with pain over those trapezius muscles, discussed in the cervical spine section, may think they have pain in the shoulder and tell their doctor so; however, true shoulder pain emanating from the multiple components of the shoulder joint is almost always referred to the *deltoid muscle* (Fig. 11). Unfortunately, once a doctor hears the word *shoulder* from the patient who believes this trapezius pain is shoulder pain, he may fail to consider that the symptoms could really be from the neck. Therefore, it is most important that you realize pains over the trapezius muscles are not from the shoulder.

To understand what can go wrong with the shoulder, we must consider its anatomy. Like the hip joint, the shoulder is a ball-and-socket joint, but it differs from the hip joint in one major way. The hip is such a stable joint that if all the structures around it were removed, a type of inherent suction within the joint would hold the ball firmly in place.

The shoulder, however, is not so stable. Its parts include a half-moon-shaped top end of upper arm bone, *head of the humerus* [HEW-mer-us];

The Shoulder

the *glenoid*, or shoulder socket, a shallow cavity in the *scapula* [SKAP-u-la], or shoulder blade (Fig. 10); and associated ligaments, tendons, and cartilage. A type of fibrous cartilage ring surrounds the entire glenoid, *glenoideum labrum* (Fig. 9). This ring is where all the ligaments attach and serves as an extension of the bony socket. With such a shallow socket, the shoulder has no negative pressure to hold its ball securely in place, leaving it relatively unstable. On the other hand, the shoulder is much more flexible than the hip. Furthermore, the ligaments of the shoulder are loose (Fig. 10), permitting a global motion of the joint, and the shoulder's only significant bony attachment to the rest of the body is through the *acromioclavicular* [ah-CHROME-ee-oh-kla-VICK-u-lar] *joint*, between the *acromion* [ah-CHROME-ee-on], a projection of the shoulder blade where it joins the end of the *clavicle* [KLAV-ickle], or collarbone (Fig. 10). Otherwise, only muscles attach the shoulder to the upper rib cage and torso. Try to visualize the shoulder blade moving on the back of the chest and the loose attachments between the ball and the shallow socket that allow motion there as well. These are essentially two centers of motion that allow the incredible flexibility found nowhere else but in the shoulder joint.

How does the shoulder joint work? The deltoid, the big muscle on the outside of the upper arm (Fig.11), covers all the structures in Figure 9. Without this muscle, which does most of the work, the shoulder couldn't function. Ligaments, loose though they may be, connect the ball to the socket, and tendons from four muscles—the subscapularis, supraspinatus, infraspinatus, and teres minor (Fig. 12A, B, and C)—from the scapula pull the ball to the socket. When the largest of these four muscles, the subscapularis [sub-sca-pu-LAIR-is] (Fig. 12A), contracts, it rotates the arm inward, in toward the body. When the other three muscles (Fig. 12B) contract, they rotate the arm outward, away from the body. Therefore, these four muscles are called *rotators*, and their combined tendons surrounding most of the ball forming a cuff-like structure. Voila—*Rotator cuff,* often mispronounced as "rotator cup" or "rotary cup." There is another tendon, the long head of the biceps (Fig.12C), about the shoulder, but it is not a part of the rotator cuff and will be discussed later.

When all these muscles contract, they set the ball against the socket and allow the deltoid muscle to lift the arm. Without these rotator cuff muscles and tendons, the deltoid couldn't lift the arm at all, and the placement of the arm in so many positions would be lost. At rest, a natural tension in these rotator muscles stabilizes the ball against the socket and keeps it from sagging, giving the shoulder a relative stability. I know I've presented a lot of medical terms here, but it's most important to comprehend them because I'll be referring to many of them. Please check back and review the figures 9, 10, and 11 when you feel you need to.

Listed below are the most common shoulder problems I saw in my practice, from the most common to the least frequent:

- Rotator cuff complaints
- Biceps-tendon problems
- Adhesive capsulitis (often called "frozen shoulder")
- Fractures or dislocations from trauma
- Injuries to or arthritis in the acromioclavicular joint
- Internal disorders, including arthritis, torn cartilage, and erosion of the socket

The Shoulder

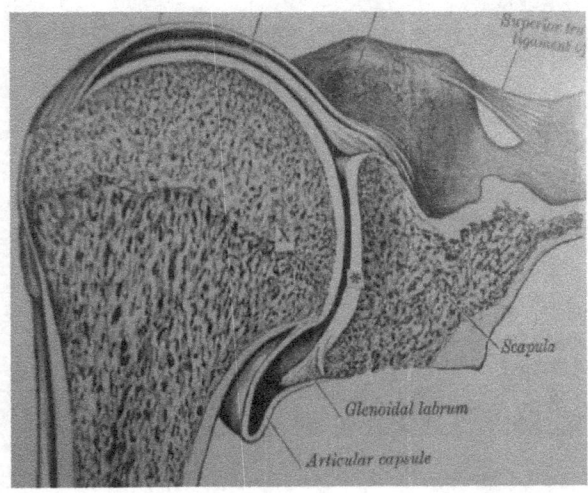

Fig. 9: Right shoulder joint: humeral head,
the ball (x), glenoid (*), and the socket
Note the Glenoideum Labrum at the bottom of the glenoid.
Gray's Anatomy, 1966

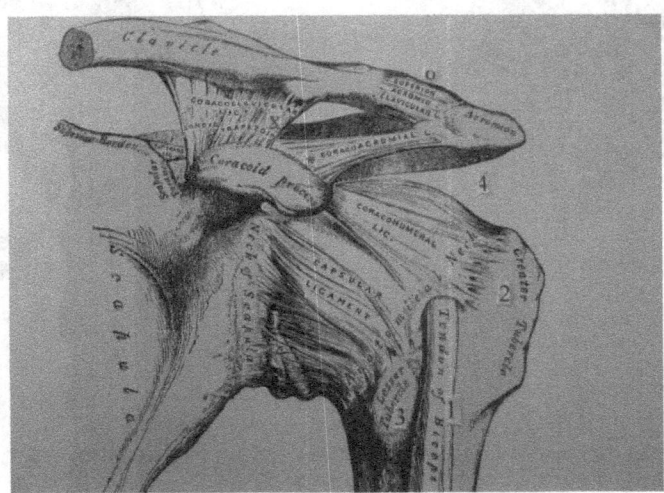

Fig. 10: Left shoulder joint with its loose ligaments; A-C joint and ligaments (o); coraco-acromial ligament (*); coraco-clavicular ligaments (x); long head of biceps (1); greater tuberosity (2) where rotator cuff tendons insert; lesser tuberosity (3) where the subscapularis tendon inserts (4); the subacromial space (4). Gray's Anatomy, 1966

The Way I See It

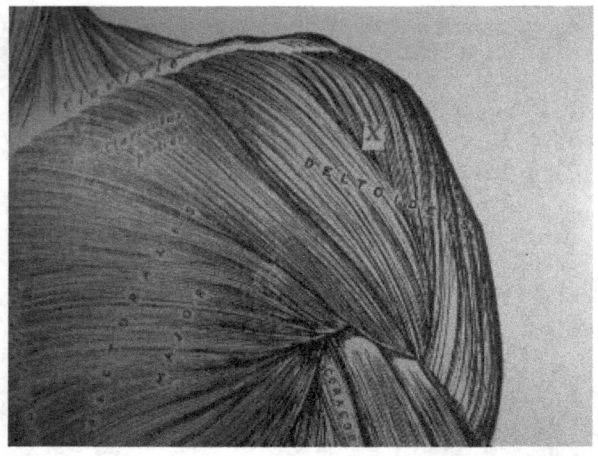

Fig. 11: Left deltoid muscle (x) covers outside of the shoulder.
Gray's Anatomy, 1966

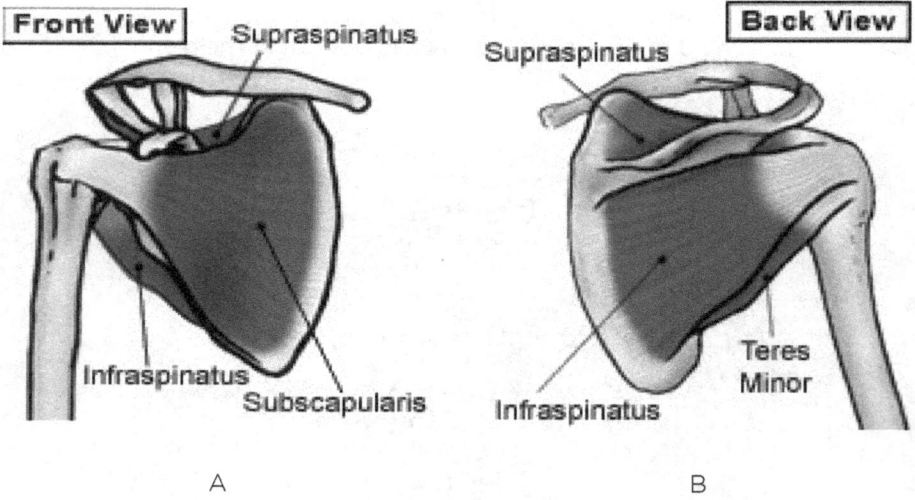

Fig. 12A: right shoulder anterior (front) view:
subscapularis muscle and its tendon inserting into lesser tuberosity (*) of the humerus.

12B: right shoulder posterior (back) view:
supraspinatus, infraspinatus, and teres minor rotator muscles
and tendons inserting into greater tuberosity (x).
www.Moore-Chiropractic.com

The Shoulder

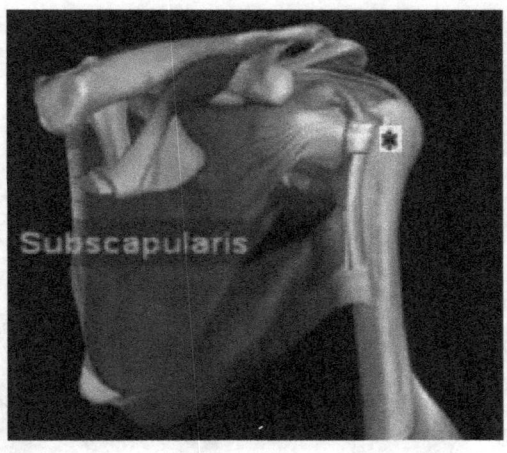

C

Fig. 12C: Note long biceps tendon covered by a thick ligament in the bicipital groove (*); Lennard Funk and www.shoulderdoc.co.uk

Degenerative and Inflammatory Conditions of the Shoulder

The Rotator Cuff

The rotator cuff tendons occupy a snug area confined above by a part of the shoulder blade known as the *acromion* (Fig. 13). This space, like many others in our bodies, contains a thin, filmy two-layered sac called a *bursa*. The rotator cuff moves more smoothly through its space beneath the acromion because of this *subacromial* [sub-ah-CHROME-ee-all], meaning "under the acromion," *bursa*. The effect is the similar to wearing two pairs of thin socks inside ski boots: the two socks glide on one another, decreasing friction and allowing less skin irritation. This subacromial bursa (Fig. 13) is one on the largest in the body, smaller only than a bursa in the hip and over the kneecap. "-*itis*" means "inflammation of." Hence, inflammation of a bursa is considered "*bursitis*."

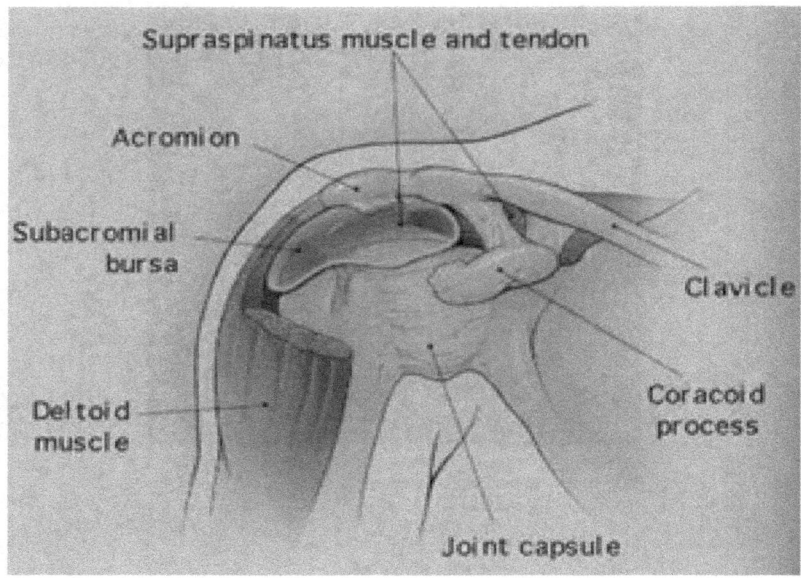

Fig. 13 : Subacromial bursa under the acromion
and on top of the rotator cuff.
www.handbook.muh.ie/rheum/Bursitis.htm

As a rule, this marvelous rotator cuff works very well, allowing lifting, throwing, catching, pushing, and pulling, but like any body part, it can wear out. The first change is usually an undetectable decrease in blood supply, possibly caused by the repetition of minimal, unnoticed injuries, a specific noticeable injury, or a natural occurrence. Quarterbacks and baseball pitchers are often diagnosed with shoulder problems involving rotator cuff injuries. In those cases, the cause is probably repetitive throwing motions. Yet far more folks with rotator cuff problems are not athletes and have never consistently thrown a ball. So why are they the ones with the most rotator cuff symptoms?

The trouble starts close to the tendons' attachment to bone onto the humerus at the greater tuberosity. For some reason, this area has few or no blood vessels even at birth. Codman[1], who discovered this condition, called it the "critical area" as he believed it was the likely site for future tendon troubles, calcification, swelling, and partial tears of these tendons. Most parts of the body need a blood supply to function, and if the blood supply is reduced or interrupted, the body almost always reacts by sending "fix-it" cells and fluid, *plasma*, to the area in question. When you burn yourself, redness, swelling, and a fluid-filled blister may occur. Something similar happens to any tendon that, suddenly or over time, loses its blood supply. Like the burned tissue, the tendon reacts with redness caused by increased blood cells and swelling as a result of an invasion of these fix-it cells, a condition we call *acute tendinitis* (*acute*, meaning it comes on suddenly).

Just as the burned area in soft tissue soon begins to heal, the affected tendon also starts to mend. The body's circulation carries the fluid and fix-it cells away, and the tendon returns to normal with a reestablished blood supply. However, in the so-called critical area, with its inherent poor or absent blood supply, healing may take longer or not occur at all. Any persistent accumulation of fluid may eventually result in scar tissue, leaving a thickened tendon, a longer-term condition sometimes called *chronic tendinitis*. The correct name for this condition is really *chronic tendinosis* since there is really no evidence of inflammation in this state, the fix-it cells being absent. *Chronic* means "permanent or long lasting," in contrast with *acute*.

In other areas of the body, an inflammatory reaction—an "-itis"— may be only a nuisance, causing little or no discomfort. But many inflammatory shoulder problems cause enough discomfort that folks seek a doctor's help. Many of these conditions come about because the blood supply to the affected area has lessened or been eliminated altogether. We have no scientific answers for why this happens, so we say the loss or reduction of blood supply is *idiopathic*, meaning "of unknown cause." Some doctors believe this failure comes on naturally, while others blame it on overuse or repeated minor injury. Most of the time, we don't know why.

But let's get back to the rotator cuff. If it swells only a little in its snug space, everyday activities such as overhead motions, lifting, pushing, pulling, and throwing may cause only discomfort over the deltoid muscle, the shoulder's usual site for referred pain. Some folks will conclude that the muscle is merely strained, so they don't see a doctor about it. But if the rotator cuff continues to be irritated and compressed, the bursa may also become secondarily inflamed, resulting in bursitis. As the bursa (Fig.13) enlarges and becomes more irregular, it rides through the tight space beneath the acromion, creating rippling noises and crunching sounds or *crepitus* [KREP-it-tus]. If the tendon is thick as well and the bursa inflamed, this subacromial space doesn't increase in size to accommodate these changes, causing even more compression, irritation, and impingement on the affected parts as one elevates his arm, known as an *impingement syndrome*.

Treatment for acute inflammation or impingement syndrome may include anti-inflammatory medications, local injections of refined steroid, wet heat, physical therapy for ultrasound, and electrical stimulation to reduce the reaction and get the bursa and tendon back to normal size. Once the condition is chronic, however, with permanent scar tissue—or *fibrosis* [fye-BRO-sis]—in both the bursa and the tendon, these treatments may help very little.

This scar tissue within the tendon is not as strong as the tendon itself. Over time, a slow, gradual splitting or fragmenting of this area may begin to weaken the tendon. It usually begins inside and works its way out from the center, mostly degenerating toward the joint side of the rotator cuff tendon, at which point we call it an *incomplete tear of the rotator cuff* (Fig. 14B). It is truly not a tear, more of a weakening or fragmentation of the tissue.

Rotator cuff disturbances can be minimal, or they can progress to create major difficulties. If fragmentation happens to progress to the top, or bursal, side of the rotator cuff, it can cause a flap-like tear that snaps back and forth with shoulder motion. Over time, the entire tendon may split, tear, and pull away from bone entirely, leaving small tendon fibers on the bone, a *complete rotator cuff tear* (Fig. 14C). The changes described above don't always result in a full thickness or complete rotator cuff tear, but because fragmented scar tissue weakens the entire tendon, a complete tear is usually the end result.

A complete tear may be small and affect only one tendon. If larger, it may affect two or three tendons and cause them to retract farther from the greater tuberosity (Fig. 14C). In that case, the muscles attached to these tendons can't function properly, but if the condition is a fairly recent development, the surgeon has a good chance of reattaching them in their original positions no matter how far they have retracted. In other cases, if the tendons have been separated from the bone for a long time, the tendon and its muscle can scar down, contract, and become almost impossible to pull back and reattach. We call these tears "massive," and many procedures are used to attempt to correct them, with varying degrees of success.

Rotator cuff tears can be diagnosed by physical exam, arthrography, and MRI (magnetic resonance imaging). My father wrote extensively on arthrography of the shoulder[2], and I was able to improve on his techniques by using X-ray fluoroscopy[3]. Nowadays, most physicians use the MRI as their diagnostic technique of choice.

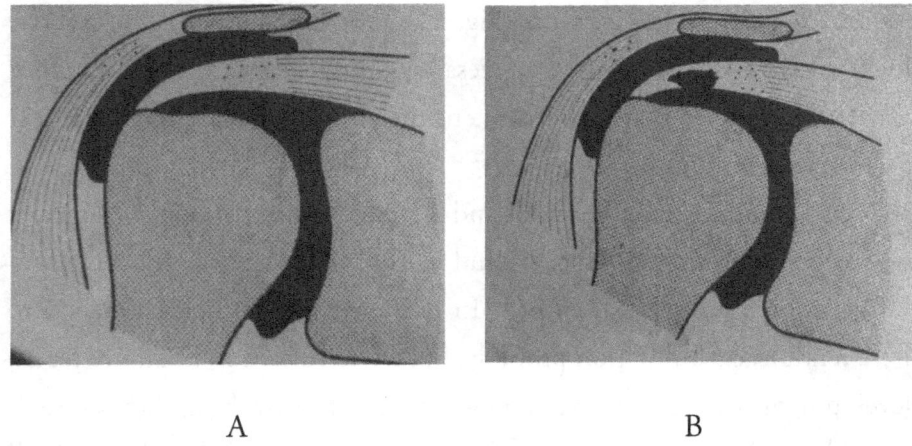

Fig. 14: A. Normal rotator cuff insertion on greater tuberosity; B. Partial rotator cuff tear.

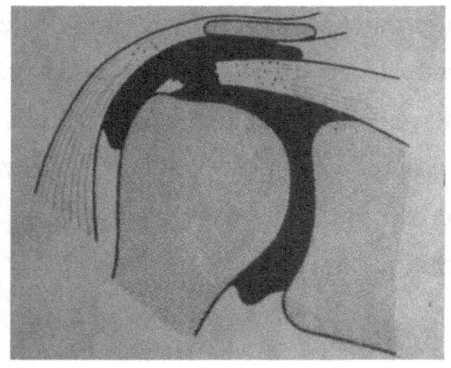

Fig. 14C: full-thickness rotator cuff tear with mild retraction. Massive tears can retract to the top of glenoid, the socket (x). Illustrations of Thomas Neviaser, MD

The initial treatment for all rotator cuff complaints is conservative: anti-inflammatory medications, wet heat, instruction in use of the arm to avoid aggravation by daily activities, and cortisone injections. When an injection is necessary, the best site is the subacromial space, where the steroid solution can soak the bursa and tendon. Injections into a space

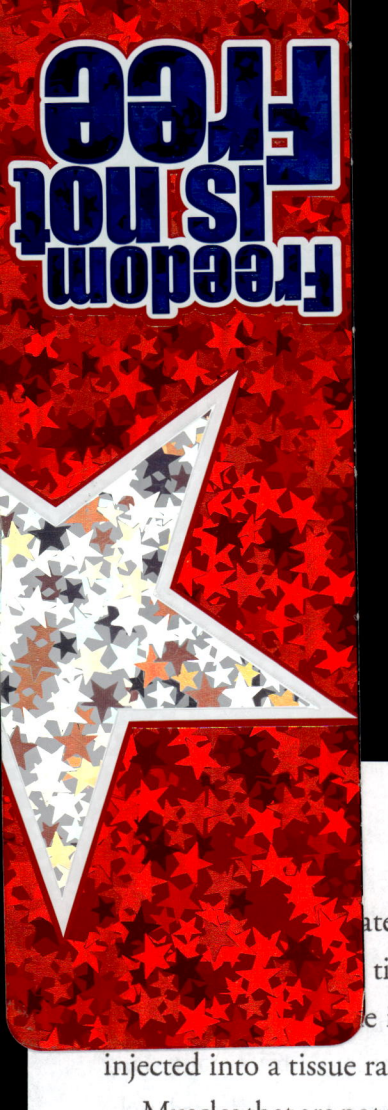

The Shoulder

...ated, with very little discomfort. On the other hand, ... tissue such as scar or thickened bursal walls will elicit ... injection is initially painful, the fluid was probably injected into a tissue rather than the subacromial space.

Muscles that are not used or used less than normal can shrink and weaken, a condition termed *disuse atrophy* [AT-trow-fee]. Any time a doctor sees a deltoid muscle that's weaker and smaller than the one on the opposite side, he should think about rotator cuff disease. Atrophy of the muscles over the shoulder blade is even more of a concern since these muscles are the ones attached to the rotator cuff tendons. The more evident the atrophy, the larger the complete tear and the less chance of an easy repair.

If the rotator cuff is not working as it should, the orthopaedic surgeon can often repair it by use of arthroscopy or with a slightly wider "open" incision (*mini-open repair*), and in some cases, an standard open repair. Results are quite good for surgery for small tears but less successful in larger tears that have become chronic.

Surprisingly, any of these conditions may occur with absolutely no pain. On the other hand, they may cause considerable pain from the start and worsen over time. Rotator cuff malfunctions follow no predictable pain pattern except that the pattern is almost always over the deltoid muscle. Tears of the same size in different patients can result in completely different intensity of complaints.

If all conservative treatments fail, surgical intervention can help, but it's important to know that without surgery, the tear may get bigger though not necessarily more painful. If you're considering having surgery for a rotator cuff tear, keep in mind that this is a major surgical procedure with known complications, and that you will need appropriate rehabilitation, including exercise and physical therapy. Your surgeon should inform you about all these factors as well as the type of surgery he plans. Before you agree to an operation of any kind, it's always a good idea to seek a second opinion.

The deciding factors in your decision about surgery should be 1) your degree of pain and 2) the extent to which the problem limits your daily activities. Other than in an emergency situation, these are good yardsticks to use when considering any orthopaedic surgery. Extreme or acute pain is not always the deciding factor, strange as it may seem. Chronic pain—not extreme, lasting for months with loss of sleep—is probably the number one reason my patients decided to undergo rotator cuff surgery. Other acceptable reasons include loss of strength and movement limited by pain.

I remember one young man, an absolute health and exercise "nut," who had a very mild case of rotator cuff tendinosis. Early inflammation of his cuff had caused an impingement syndrome. He felt pain only with certain motions during exercise and had no other symptoms or night pain, yet he decided to have the surgery even though I tried for six months to talk him out of it.

After the surgery, he was a happy camper for a while, but six months later, he was back complaining of discomfort. His symptoms then were milder than before the surgery, and when he asked me to operate on his shoulder again I refused, telling him that it could make the condition worse, and that it made more sense to avoid scarring the tendon by modifying his exercise program. He never understood and never returned for follow-up. I didn't think this man's lifestyle was affected enough to warrant another operation, but he thought otherwise. Everyone has his own personal definition of lifestyle disturbance, no matter how small.

At surgery, the ends of a fragmented or torn rotator cuff are trimmed back to healthy tissue and sutured back into the area of freshly prepared boney groove where the tendons originally inserted. This is done with sutures through the groove in the bone or by using metal or bio-absorbable bone anchors through which the sutures are placed. As mentioned, this can be accomplished with a pure arthroscopic procedure performed through multiple small incisions, a mini-open approach in combination with arthroscopy, or a purely open technique. Your physician will describe the technique that works best for him.

When repairing a rotator cuff, I believe in enlarging the subacromial space for better visualization as well as allowing a larger area for the repaired cuff to move and heal. Remember how the rotator cuff lives in a snug space? That's the subacromial space—the space between the humeral head and the acromion (Fig. 9, #4). When a tendon thickens or partially or fully fragments, this space can scarcely contain its bulk, and further irritation occurs, especially when the arm is moved away from the body. To correct this condition, the surgeon may release or altogether remove a dense, wide ligament on the front of the acromion that covers part of the rotator cuff and shave the undersurface of the acromion itself to enlarge the space. This operation, known as an *acromioplasty* [uh-CHROME-ee-oh-plasty], may be done either arthroscopically or as an open procedure. Again, there will be some oozing of blood here, establishing another site in which scar tissue may later form postoperatively.

So how successful is rotator cuff surgery? Every surgeon has his own statistics, and because rotator cuff disease comes in varying degrees and forms, there is probably no one answer. If we include all rotator cuff conditions ranging from tendinosis and impingement syndrome to massive tears, I would say surgery is probably 80–85 percent successful. Massive tears are very difficult to repair, sometimes necessitating grafts, tendon transfers, and more than one operation, but fortunately such tears are few and far between. Even though results of surgery for massive tears may be only good to excellent in less than 35 percent of cases, the more common and less complicated procedures for rotator cuff disease increase the overall statistics of success.

What complications can occur as a result of the surgery? Major ones are listed below:

- Anesthetic complications
- Bacterial infection
- Re-tearing of the tendon repair during rehabilitation
- Failure of the repair to heal, with later re-tearing
- Loss of motion and pain caused by scar tissue from the surgery itself
- Continued pain
- Weakness

The first three speak for themselves. As for the fourth, once repaired, why wouldn't the tendon heal?

First, the area of bone from which the tendon originally tore is the area to which it must be reattached. I believe the initial loss of blood supply to the tendon often occurs here, at the bone-tendon interface. Multiple biopsies of bone in this area proved to me that, in most instances, the bone had no blood supply, and sometimes, it was even *sclerotic* [skler-OTT-ick], or hard and dead. Despite the surgeon's best effort, an area that is that unhealthy may never regain an adequate blood supply to allow healing.

Secondly, the tendon may have weakened and pulled apart because it, too, had a poor blood supply or none, and while the surgeon must trim away all unhealthy tendon tissue, the tendon that's left may not be healthy enough to heal. In addition, if the tendon is cut back too far in the effort to reach healthy tendon, reattaching it to bone may create so much tension that the tendon may pull out and retract again after the operation. As you can see, the operation is not easy to perform successfully every time.

After I made tendon repairs on my patients, I insisted they wear an *immobilizer* for three weeks, keeping the hand and arm pointing straight ahead rather than across the chest. I felt that letting the arm rest in a sling across the chest allowed the postoperative scar tissue to occur in the most inappropriate position thereby causing a longer rehabilitation for my patients.

What happens after the sling is removed is as important as the operation itself. Before the surgery, I always took time to teach my patients how to do the *passive-motion exercises* they would need to begin three weeks after the operation. It was important for them to know ahead of time how to do these exercises because many folks have trouble grasping them and needed practice to prepare. After I instructed them, I had them practice with me observing to be sure they understood.

With passive-motion exercises, the arm is moved about but without using the shoulder muscles connected to the repaired tendons. The person is taught to bend from the waist, which relieves tension on the tendon repair, and sway the body to swing the totally limp arm forward and backward like a pendulum and then in a circular motion. Another passive-motion exercise calls for a rope-and-pulley system. With this method, the patient grasps the rope's handle with the hand on the same side as the repaired shoulder, keeping the shoulder limp, and uses the opposite arm to pull the affected arm up and down (Fig. 15).

Still another method calls for lying on one's back, holding a short pole or stick with both hands pointed at the ceiling and, using the opposite arm, pushing or rotating the operated arm into an externally rotated (outward) position.

I always told my patients that once they completed their exercises, they should make a habit of keeping their hand on the operated side in a pocket rather than holding the arm across the chest. I stressed this because most people instinctively hold the affected arm across the chest to protect it and avoid any pain, but as scar tissue develops, motion can be severely restricted in this position. This is also why I immobilized the arm in a neutral position after surgery. Patients' rehabilitation times were substantially reduced with this.

Remember, surgery always involves some bleeding—not massive, just an inevitable slight oozing during the operation and for a short time afterward—so the resultant clotted blood eventually becomes scar tissue or fibrosis. Once that happens, if the arm is held too still across the chest, the scar tissue becomes rigid and tight, limiting motion away from the body and causing pain, somewhat like a rubbery glue that gives when stretched but draws back to its original length afterward. So if long periods pass without moving the arm from the cross-chest position, that rigid scar tissue will cause moving the arm freely in all directions difficult, if not impossible.

After three weeks in the immobilizer, followed by nine more weeks of only passive-motion exercises, I had my patients begin active motions and exercises to strengthen the shoulder muscles. With active motion, the patient is encouraged to strengthen the shoulder muscles and regain a full range of motion by using those muscles. There's no point in continuing to protect the surgical area because if the repair hasn't healed after three months, protecting it further will usually be useless.

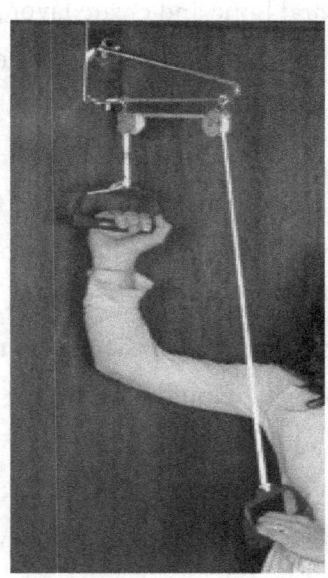

Fig.15. Rope and pulley for passive range of motion for the right shoulder. The left hand pulls down on the rope, lifting the limp right arm.

For anyone with bone and joint problems, specific types of exercise are often necessary before or after surgery. Many folks think the resultant pain from these exercises means something is wrong, so they might stop the exercises, believing they're protecting the area and avoiding making matters worse. Stretching of the body's tissues or scar tissue can cause pain; however, if properly done, these exercises *hurt but will not harm.*

When instructing someone in a passive-motion exercise program, I always made it clear that these exercises were necessary to stretch the scar tissue and keep it from becoming rigid. In addition, I told them that although the stretching would hurt, as the scar tissue loosened, the pain would decrease. The tighter the scar tissue, the more pain the stretching causes, but such exercises are essential for a full recovery.

While the function of the exercises is to keep the arm useful, they play no part in the actual healing. The surgeon's aims are to establish a blood supply between tendon and bone and create favorable conditions to return the bursa to a healthy state. If all this happens, the operation is considered a success. Factors that can work against success include overzealous exercising, beginning active motion or lifting the arm against resistance too soon, and re-injuring the joint. If any of these happen, the tendon may tear or pull out again. The surgeon may have made his very best effort, but there will always be folks who, knowingly or unknowingly, decide that being pain-free means the surgery cured them, so they begin moving the affected arm too actively and sabotage what would have been a good result.

I remember a young lady in her late thirties with a relatively small rotator cuff tear of her right shoulder. At breakfast six weeks after her operation, she accidentally knocked over a coffeepot and impulsively reached out to catch it. The repaired tendon pulled out, and she underwent a second operation. The result of the repeat surgery was so good that she returned several years later for the same repair to her left shoulder, and six weeks after her second surgery, she slipped in the shower and reached out to catch herself with her left hand. This re-tear also required another operation, again with a happy result. She and I were certainly thankful she had only two shoulders.

Lack of pain after surgery doesn't necessarily mean everything is healed. Folks who fail to follow the surgeon's instructions after a rotator cuff repair may well need repeat operations, and most second rotator cuff surgeries can be less successful than the first. I had to constantly remind my patients that following the proper rehabilitation program was essential for a good result.

Degeneration similar to that taking place in the rotator cuff can also affect the *long head of the biceps* (Fig. 9 [3 and 4]), a tendon of the *biceps muscle* in the front of the upper arm that originates inside the shoulder joint and is very closely related to the rotator cuff. This tendon, too, may become inflamed and swell with compression and irritation in its confined space, leading to partial fragmentation or tearing and eventual rupture.

The biceps muscle consists of two distinct bundles, giving it its name, which means "two heads" in Latin. The *long tendon head of the biceps* and the *short head of the biceps* muscle (Fig. 16) originate in different areas around the shoulder. The long head is the smaller of the two. For now, we'll concern ourselves only with the long head.

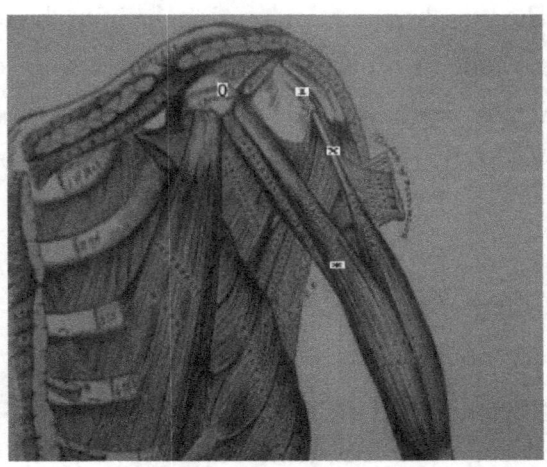

Fig. 16 : The left biceps muscle: notice the long-head tendon (x) entering the joint (1), whereas the short head (*) originates at the coracoid process (O); the bicipital groove covered by thick ligament (1).
Gray's Anatomy, 1966

The long-head tendon begins inside the shoulder joint at the top of the socket and emerges from the shoulder through a groove in the humerus to meet the long muscle head midway along the upper arm. This groove is covered by a thick ligament that confines the long-head tendon to a tight tunnel for a short distance (Fig. 16). An extension of the *synovium* [sin-NO-vee-um] of the shoulder joint covers the biceps tendon. The synovium secretes *synovial fluid* that lubricates the joint and helps to nourish the cartilage covering the bones that form the shoulder joint and the biceps tendon as well.

If the rotator cuff is degenerating enough, the synovium in the joint reacts and thickens. It does not produce its normal fluid and will secrete other substances that may hasten tendon degeneration. The long-head tendon is especially affected in its confined space outside the joint (Fig. 16), in the groove under the thick ligament quite a distance from the joint. Pain from this condition is often similar to pain from the rotator cuff, and if the surgeon fails to remove the synovial covering of the tendon or explore the portion of the long-head tendon outside the joint, he will not discover a possible biceps tendon problem that may be causing some, if not all, of the patient's pain. Failure to detect this trouble spot before or during surgery may leave the patient with some of the preoperative pain after the operation.

Calcific Tendinitis of the Rotator Cuff

Loss of blood supply to the so-called critical area isn't the only thing that causes degeneration and fragmentation of the rotator cuff. A chemical change can also bring on difficulties. If the pH (the measure of the acidity or alkalinity of fluid and tissue) of this area becomes acidic enough, probably as a result of the ongoing degenerative process, calcium can invade the tendon, causing acute inflammation and swelling to accommodate the calcium deposit (Fig. 17). As the calcium is deposited, increasing pressure inside the tendon causes a great deal of pain with the slightest shoulder motion, this pain again being referred to the deltoid muscle. I have seen some of the toughest people cry with this condition because it is almost impossible for them to find a comfortable position as the pressure within the tendon increases.

Because the ballooning of the tendon is the problem, a doctor can insert a needle into the tendon to let the thick, liquefied calcium escape and relieve the pressure, which will reduce or eliminate the pain. Adding a local anesthetic and a refined steroid to bathe the painful area will also give relief down the road.

If not all the calcium can be removed by the needling technique and pain continues, arthroscopic surgery to make a small incision in the tendon and remove the calcium deposit may be necessary. You might think that would leave the tendon with a defect, but the space previously occupied by calcium rapidly fills with blood supplied by the bursa, fibrous tissue results, and the tendon heals.

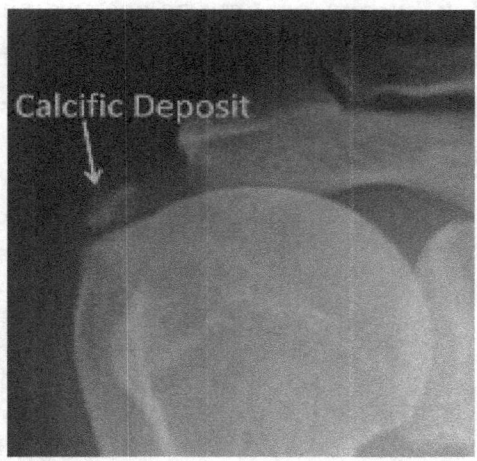

Fig. 17. Calcium deposit in the "critical area" of supraspinatus tendon at its insertion to bone
www.shoulderdoc.co.uk

Acromioclavicular Separation

Remember that the shoulder is mostly attached to the body by muscles and only a single joint, the acromioclavicular joint (Fig. 9) where the acromion portion of the shoulder blade joins the end of the collarbone. It's this joint—and not the actual ball-and-socket shoulder joint—that's disrupted when athletes suffer a "separated shoulder." In this joint, like every other, a special cartilage covers both ends of the bones that form the joint while a small crescent structure, a *meniscus* [men-NISS-cuss] (*meniscus* meaning "crescent"), lies between the bone ends inside the joint.

When the acromioclavicular joint separates, ligaments associated with it can rupture, the most drastic and common separation being labeled grade 3. The causative injury may be a severe blow, or it may occur when someone lands on the top of the shoulder. This downward force on the acromion and the shoulder blade will rupture several ligaments, and immediately afterward, the end of the collarbone may ride higher than its normal position in relation to the acromion (Fig. 18). This injury can be left alone without surgery, or it can be operated on at any time after the injury. The shoulder usually won't lose any motion or strength, and weakness may not be noticeable unless there is pain, in which case surgery is probably advisable.

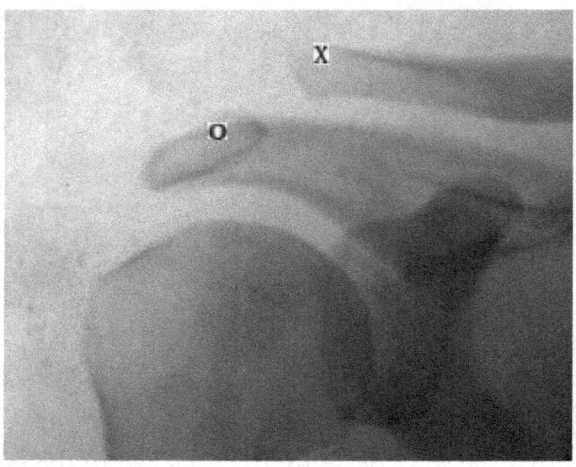

Fig.18: Acromioclavicular separation, grade 3; the end of the clavicle (x) riding far above the acromion (o).

Acromioclavicular Arthritis

The acromioclavicular joint (AC joint) is probably one of the first joints to undergo arthritic changes. I have seen X-ray evidence of severe arthritic changes in this joint in people between twenty and thirty years of age. So much force is placed on this joint that it's no wonder that it degenerates relatively early in life. Often, these changes don't cause pain, but when they do, it's usually directly over the joint. At times, the pain can also be referred back over the clavicle to the top of the trapezius muscle. This is another situation that can lead to confusion for the doctor who may believe the pain is coming from the neck.

If there's a painful arthritis in this joint, it will always be tender when examined, no matter where its pain is referred. In the course of a physical examination, therefore, the doctor should always press on the top of the acromioclavicular joint. One important test can help narrow down the possible sources of the pain if the AC joint is suspected: an injection of the anesthetic Lidocaine into the joint. This little joint can hold only a small amount of fluid, and if the injection does not relieve the pain, one must look elsewhere for the cause. If the local anesthetic entirely relieves the pain, this joint is definitely the cause of pain.

Once arthritis in the acromioclavicular joint is diagnosed, if conservative treatment fails, and the pain is enough to disturb the patient's lifestyle, it's time to consider surgery to widen the joint to keep the bones from rubbing together. This procedure is called an acromioclavicular *arthroplasty* (*arthroplasty* simply meaning "an operation on a joint"). When the acromioclavicular joint is the sole cause of shoulder pain, this procedure—either arthroscopic or open—is highly successful, with few complications. The surgeon removes a small section of the end of the clavicle. This is the procedure of choice for isolated acromioclavicular arthritis.

I first performed this operation arthroscopically in the 1990s, something that wasn't generally done at the time. One of my patients generously allowed me to operate on him through the arthroscope. The surgery was relatively easy, and the result was most satisfying to both the patient and me. However, the hardest portion of the surgery was his tattoo. He had tattoos over his entire body, and because his favorite one lay directly over the affected joint, my greatest challenge was choosing the appropriate spots for the small incisions to avoid deforming the tattoo.

Acromioclavicular arthritis can occur by itself, or it can be associated with rotator cuff disease. Arthritic changes of the joint often form *osteophytes* [OSS-tee-oh-fights], or bone spurs (Fig. 19), that can protrude into the subacromial space, irritating the rotator cuff underneath. Failure to look for and correct such conditions in the course of repairing a rotator cuff may leave the patient with continued pain. Widening the joint surgically eliminates the bone spurs and does not interfere with the mechanics of shoulder motion.

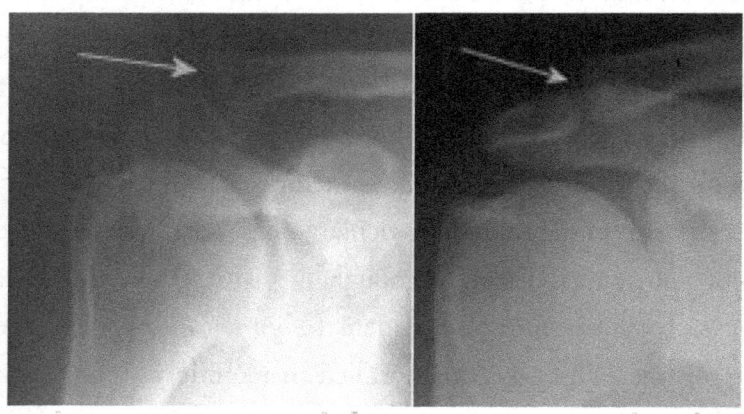

Fig. 19: AC arthritis, left, with joint narrowing and bone spurs (left of 1); normal AC joint on right for comparison.
www.shoulderdoc.co.uk

Dislocations of the Shoulder

Because of its basic instability, the shoulder joint is more apt to dislocate than any other joint. With the most common dislocation, *anterior* (meaning "in front") (Fig. 20), the ball is forced completely out in front of the socket. If the ball is driven out the back of the joint, that's considered a *posterior dislocation* which is far less common.

With a *partial* anterior dislocation—a *subluxation* [sub-LUX-a-shun]—the ball does not fully dislocate and pops back into place. Both a subluxation and a full dislocation can result from a fall onto an outstretched arm, driving the arm up and back so that the ball is thrust against the front of the socket. Most full dislocations can be remedied only by *reduction* (manipulation into correct position either by the patient or someone else), to replace the ball in its socket, whereas subluxations always reduce themselves.

Both a subluxation and a full dislocation will disrupt the same soft tissues inside the joint. Ligaments that attach to the ball arise from the *gleniodeum labrum,* a small ridge of tissue that surrounds the socket (Fig. 21). An anterior dislocation or subluxation will partially rip the labrum and its ligaments away from the bony socket's edge in front. The resulting permanent looseness of these structures means that certain movements or positions of the shoulder can result in *recurrent* or *habitual* subluxations or dislocations in the future.

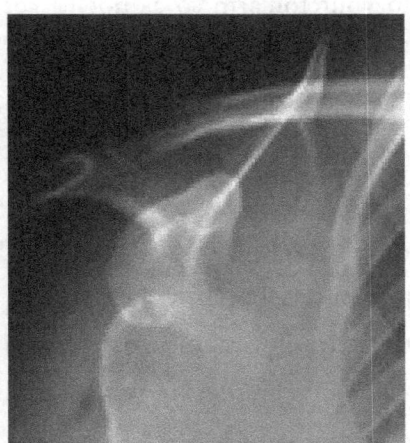 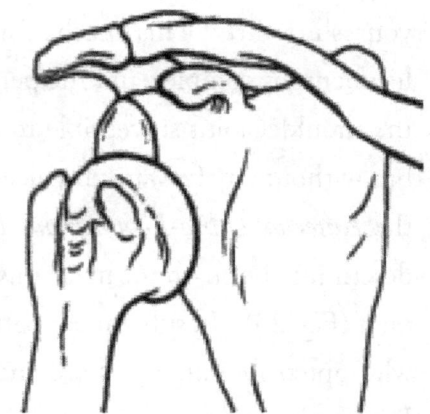

Fig 20: X-ray and diagram of dislocation, anterior, shoulder: ball totally in front of socket.

This injury was first described by the German physician Perthes in a publication in the late 1800s[6]. The publication never was distributed widely, and this pathology was not well-known until an Englishman,

Bankart, published his findings in the 1920s[7]. Since that time, the labral/ligamentous avulsion occurring with an anterior dislocation as described above has been known as a *Bankart lesion* (Fig. 22). The back of the ball is almost always compressed on the front edge of the socket, causing a compression fracture of the back of the ball in the shape of a wedge and known as a *Hill-Sachs* lesion (Fig. 24). This locks the ball out of the joint thereby necessitating a maneuvering of the arm to replace the ball in opposition to the socket. If the ball is driven out the back of the joint, it is known as a *posterior dislocation*, a condition much less common. A Hill-Sachs lesion can develop on the front part of the ball in these posterior cases.

In 1993, I described a variant of the Bankart lesion never before identified. I noticed the labrum and its ligaments actually slid down the front side or neck of the glenoid socket along with the lining of the bone, the *periosteum*, like a sleeve you'd slide up your forearm so as not to get your shirt dirty. This mechanism of injury displaced the entire labro-ligamentous complex and the periosteum, leaving the ligaments loose and the shoulder joint susceptible to dislocation similar to the Bankart lesion but without any forward dispalcement of the complex. I named the lesion the *Anterior Labro-Ligamentous Periosteal Sleeve Avulsion (ALPSA) lesion*, describing the anatomic mechanism of injury rather than placing my name on it (Fig. 23)[8]. In subsequent patients with recurrent dislocating shoulders who opted for surgery, those anterior sockets not presenting with a true Bankart lesion were explored and found to have a chronic ALPSA lesion in its original displaced position but covered by dense scar tissue that visually looked like the original labrum. This was the reason that, for so many decades, orthopaedists were led to believe the ligaments had ruptured and left the labrum intact. Now most surgeons know of the ALPSA lesion and appropriately correct it, allowing for many more successful repairs than in the past.

Surgery is usually necessary to prevent recurrent dislocations. In the past, various open procedures were used for the purpose, some of them designed to restrict the shoulder's ability to rotate outward. The problem here was that the anatomic disruption that led to the dislocation was never addressed. Nowadays, the surgeon will attempt to recreate the anatomy by replacing the labrum and its ligaments in their original anatomic positions, often by arthroscopic repair, and the results are very close to those derived from the open techniques of the past, with less tissue damage and equal return of normal motion.

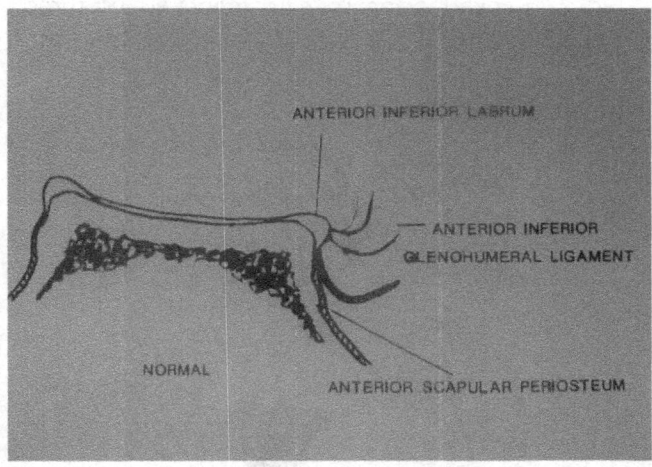

Fig. 21: Cross section of a normal glenoid, anterior labrum and ligaments attached.

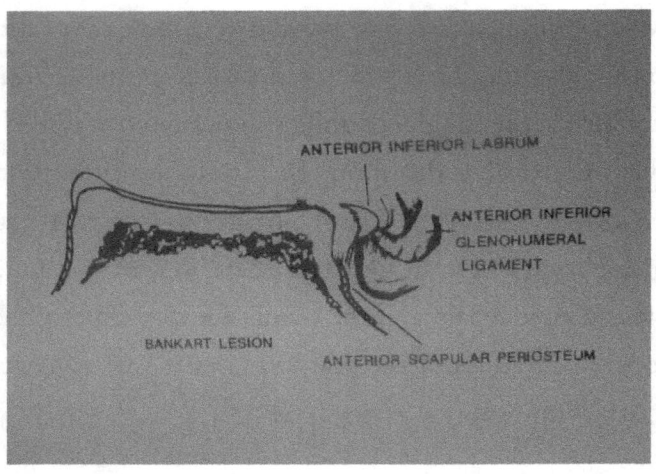

Fig. 22: Bankart lesion: note ligaments are ruptured

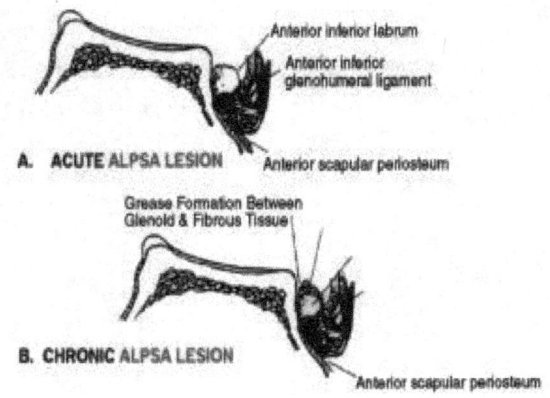

Fig. 23A: Acute ALPSA lesion: note there are no ruptured ligaments

23B: Chronic ALPSA lesion: note fibrous tissue on top of labrum

The GLAD Lesion

This is another previously undescribed defect or lesion I was able to identify in 1993, along with its mechanism of injury[9]. (Yes, 1993 was a productive year for me.) An eighteen-year-old quarterback for a local high school suffered a painful injury to his shoulder while running to his right and suddenly throwing to his left across his body without changing the direction of his torso. Subsequently, his pain subsided, but it continually recurred when throwing. At surgery, his labrum proved to be torn but not displaced, and a corresponding fraying of the hyaline cartilage covering the glenoid socket next to the labral tear was identified. I probed the labrum, and it was indeed fragmented but not detached as with a Bankart lesion or an ALPSA lesion. I actually saw several cases of GLAD lesions that year, and all the patients gave a history of their arms being forced across their chests. Surgically, these defects were smoothed off and allowed to heal for three months, and most of the patients were allowed to continue their sports.

My gut feeling is that these injuries may be a cause of shoulder arthritis in later years. In someone who had such an injury and never sought medical advice, the glenoid socket could have continued to fragment and degenerate, its deterioration eventually evolving into arthritis of the shoulder. This is speculation on my part, however, by the time I retired from active practice, none of my young patients who had socket damage were older than twenty-five.

Shoulder Arthritis

No one really knows what causes osteoarthritis of the shoulder (*osteo* means "of the bone"), which is an uncommon condition. An injury can cause it, but in the absence of any history of an injury, an inflammatory disease such as rheumatoid arthritis, or other less common disorders, it's impossible to be sure of the cause.

First of all, all bony ends forming joints are covered with *hyaline cartilage,* its purpose being to allow bones to smoothly glide on one another and give a cushioning effect. Hyaline cartilage is akin to the gristle that easily separates from a chicken bone end. It is usually somewhat firm, glistening, and white. It derives its nourishment from the fluid produced by the joint lining, the *synovium*.

What happens when the shoulder and other joints begin to degenerate? This process might be genetically programmed, but I believe it starts with the joint lining, which reacts to an injury, a microfracture, or repeated minute trauma in a specific way. This reaction leads to *synovitis* [sign-oh-VITE-tus], inflammation and swelling of the lining. Thereafter, the lining produces fluid at an increased rate, and this fluid, instead of doing its usual job of nourishing the cartilage over the bone ends, carries abnormal enzymes that actually inhibit nourishment of the cartilage.

Over time, the smooth, glistening cartilage begins to crack and fragment, losing its ability to survive. This increased fragmentation and fraying of the cartilage surface, called *chondromalacia* [con-dro-ma-LAY-she –uh], resembles the ragged end of a stick that's been dragged along the ground. As the fraying progresses, microscopic pieces break away acting as foreign bodies. The joint lining reacts by absorbing these small pieces, producing more inflammation and more abnormal fluid. At first, small fragments detach, then larger ones, partially and fully; some of them floating freely inside the joint and causing it to lock or give way.

Over the years, many areas of the joints eventually lose their cartilage covering altogether, leaving only exposed bone in a joint, and grinding and crepitus can be heard and felt. Eventually, the bones lose their ability to fit together well, causing deformity, and even more loss of motion.

In the shoulder, which is held together by muscle forces, the ball sometimes becomes deformed and is forced backward out of alignment with the socket, causing pain and loss of motion. Arthroscopic surgery to remove all loose material from the joint and shave and cauterize the diseased synovium may reduce pain for a while, but eventually, the ball-and-socket components may have to be replaced by *a prosthesis*, or artificial substitute, in an operation called *total shoulder replacement*. In the original version of this operation, a metallic ball atop a stem implanted in the upper arm bone replaced the damaged ball, and a polyethylene plastic socket replaced the deteriorated socket (Fig. 25).

However, a newer method calls for a replacement ball screwed into the bony socket and a new socket atop a stem implanted in the upper arm bone (Fig. 26). Because the newer total shoulder replacements are believed to be more stable, they are used for unstable joints and situations where the rotator cuff has greatly deteriorated. New developments come along every year, and total shoulder replacement is still evolving.

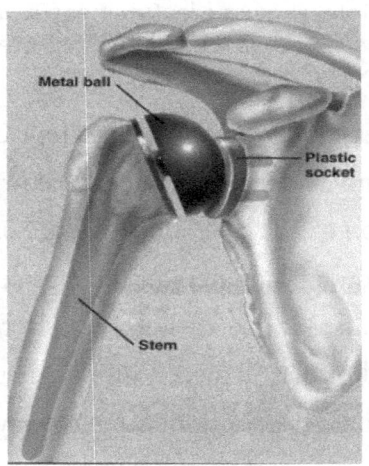

Fig. 25 : Total shoulder replacement diagram:
Metal ball with stem within the upper humerus and plastic socket on glenoid.
University Orthopedic Center, Hackensack, PA, N.J. website

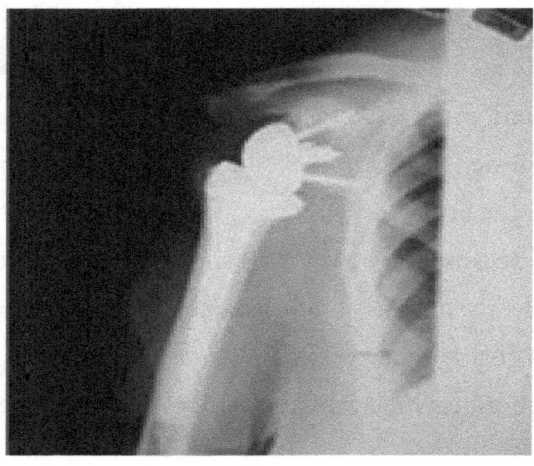

Fig. 26: Total shoulder replacement; reverse type, with socket on ball side and ball on the socket side

The main complications of total shoulder replacement surgery include anesthetic risks (as with all surgeries), superficial or deep infections (again a possible complication of any operation), failure of soft tissue repair, and dislocation, subluxation, or loosening of the replacement parts.

Deep infections must be treated immediately because if bacteria find their way to the metal or plastic pieces, they settle there and wreak havoc, unreachable by antibiotic medication. Surgery may be necessary to drain the infection, remove the prosthetic devices, or both.

Occasionally, repairs to soft tissue and tendons performed at the end of a total shoulder replacement may fail and require another operation. Pullout of a particular tendon—the *subscapularis* [sub-skap-YOU-lair-us]—is the most common, and unhealthy tissue and postoperative overexertion are the main causes. Newer surgical approaches to the shoulder have reduced the chances of this complication.

Partial and full dislocations can occur, requiring reduction, immobilization, and possible revision of the total shoulder replacement. Over time, the bone around the metal and plastic replacement parts can also gradually shrink away and cause the implants to loosen. This loosening, sometimes detectable only by X-ray, may or may not cause pain. If the pain from loosening is severe enough, another operation may be needed to revise these parts.

Adhesive Capsulitis (Frozen Shoulder)

Adhesive Capsulitis is a condition with which I have a great deal of experience.[10] It was first described by my father, Julius S. Neviaser.[11] It's sometimes called frozen shoulder, but this generic label fails to explain what's happening inside the joint or why. The name he gave it provides two facts about the disease—*adhesive*, to explain its adherent properties; and *capsulitis*, to indicate inflammation in the *joint capsule* (the ligamentous lining enveloping the shoulder joint). Its cause is unknown. Some believe it to be of an autoimmune nature. Its initial symptoms are similar to those of rotator cuff disease, including gradual onset of pain and loss of shoulder motion, but it differs from rotator cuff disease in one very important way. Usually, over the course of about nine to twelve months, the symptoms of adhesive capsulitis will diminish and eventually disappear, with no lingering after-effects. We call this type of process "self-limiting."

Adhesive capsulitis is more common in women than in men and strikes between the ages thirty-five and fifty-five. Diabetic patients are more severely hindered by this disease often not regaining all their motion, even after the process has ended. The initial mild discomfort gradually progresses to frank pain on any shoulder movement, followed by a decreasing ability to move the shoulder with even more pain. Any time folks complain of no longer being able place an arm behind the back as far as the opposite side, it should raise the doctor's suspicion of adhesive capsulitis although this isn't an infallible clue.

In 1995, I saw an unusually large number of folks with this problem who gained little or no benefit from exercises. The usual treatment was to anesthetize the patient to manipulate the shoulder and break up the adhesions in the hope of improving the range of movement. Before undertaking this manipulation, I used an arthroscope to see what was going on inside these joints and was soon able to identify three stages of the disease process. I wanted to present my findings in a paper,[11] with videotapes showing these never witnessed changes. In searching through my patient records for a normal shoulder to include as a contrast to these affected joints, I ran across the case of a nurse I had operated on for rotator cuff impingement syndrome. As I watched the tape of her operation, rather than seeing a normal joint, I saw some very early changes that I hadn't previously recognized as abnormal. Comparing this video with affected joints proved to me that this was the first stage of the disease, never before identified. After her operation, the woman continued to display undeniable signs of adhesive capsulitis that made her rehabilitation difficult. I then understood that this first stage of Adhesive Capsulitis definitely mimics the symptoms of rotator cuff tendinosis and impingement, a fact that all physicians treating shoulder problems should now realize.

On physical examination, loss of shoulder motion is apparent in any patient in the second, third, and fourth stages of this disease. In stage 2, pain accompanies any attempt to move the shoulder, with less pain in stage 3 and still less in stage 4. Patients in stage 1 may have no loss of motion, but if the patient holds the arm by his side as the doctor rotates the arm outward, the patient will often allow the arm to move only bit by bit, a series of gradual releases I call "cogwheeling." The difference between this and movement of a normal shoulder is very subtle, but an experienced doctor can detect this characteristic motion, in which case Adhesive Capsulitis must be considered.

To make sure he's dealing with Adhesive Capsulitis and not rotator cuff disease alone, the doctor should first offer the usual conservative treatment as previously described and let a month or two pass. If a gradual loss of motion becomes evident, with a decrease in all shoulder motions—including moving the arm away from the side, moving the arm across the chest, and rotating the arm up and out with the hand pointing to the ceiling—the patient probably has stage 2 Adhesive Capsulitis. On the other hand, if time passes and motion is not reduced, Adhesive Capsulitis can be ruled out and more active treatment for rotator cuff disease can begin. Making the diagnosis of rotator cuff disease without investigating the possibility of Adhesive Capsulitis can lead to a prolonged and misguided course of treatment. If an orthopaedic surgeon operates for rotator cuff disease in the face of Adhesive Capsulitis, there will be more problems afterward, and rehabilitation will be difficult and prolonged.

The usual treatment for this disease is to encourage the patient to use the shoulder and exercise the shoulder in specific directions, all to keep what motion the patient has or improve it until the process subsides. Here, pain will hurt but will not harm the patient whatsoever. An aggressive exercise program is instituted until full range of motion is obtained. Many patients can easily become unhappy because of the continued pain and loss of motion even though they have been religious in performing their exercises. The process itself may take nine months or longer. I usually saw my patients every three to four weeks, both for documenting their progress as well as giving them encouragement to continue working on their motion and assuaging their fears of never getting better.

CHAPTER 5
THE COLLARBONE (CLAVICLE)

I know I said I wasn't going to discuss fractures, but because the *clavicle* [KLAV-ic-kull], or collarbone, is the most fractured bone in the body, I decided to include it.

The clavicle is an S-shaped bone, its medial end (that portion toward the center of the body) joining the upper *sternum* or chest bone to form the *sternoclavicular* [sterno-kla-VICK-ular] *joint*. Its other end—the lateral end (the portion that is away from the center of the body)—joins the *acromion*, a portion of the *scapula* (shoulder blade) to form the *acromoclavicular joint* discussed in the last chapter.

The most common collarbone fracture results from a blow to the tip of the shoulder such as sustained with a fall when someone lands on the shoulder, exerting direct force on the bone's outside end. This force may fracture the collarbone at its outer end, in the middle or midshaft area, or both. A midshaft fracture often breaks upward, forward, or both with an obvious deformity. The fracture may be *transverse* (straight across), *oblique* (at an angle), or *comminuted* ([COM-in-noo-ted], meaning "multiple pieces").

At the moment the collarbone breaks, one will often hear a crack or pop and feel sudden pain, but even more disconcerting is the awareness

The Collarbone (Clavicle)

that the broken pieces are rubbing together. This sensation, which can persist for weeks after the fracture, is quite normal and no cause for worry. Having had two clavicle fractures myself, I'm personally familiar with this grinding sensation. With a comminuted fracture, a piece of bone may poke up under the skin, compromising its integrity, though this is rare. The problem should be dealt with surgically by making a small incision to remove all or a portion of the offending bony piece and then closing the incision to let the fracture heal on its own.

Most collarbone fractures can be treated conservatively by having the patient wear a sling or, if the fracture is displaced, a figure-eight bandage holding the shoulders back for several weeks. This treatment does not set the fracture but stretches the lining around the bone in an attempt to decrease the motion at the fracture site like a Chinese finger trap. Most of these fractures will heal on their own, but some will need to be operated on. If the surgeon believes an operation is needed, he should discuss the pros and cons with the patient. I'm not a big fan of operating on clavicle fractures as a very high percentage of them will heal on their own, even those causing an obvious deformity. Whatever malformation appears at the time of the fracture will usually persist after healing and may in fact even be slightly larger because of new bone formation at the fracture site.

Overall, orthopaedists don't usually "set" or manipulate fractures to realign the collarbone but leave them to heal as is. Recently, however, more surgeons prefer treating fractures surgically, applying plates and screws to create a more stable construct for healing and a more acceptable alignment. As with any operation for a fracture, infections and *non-unions* (failure of the fragments to unite) may occur. It was always my policy to let the fracture heal and then deal with any problems later. Non-unions of clavicles occur without surgery as well, but the percentages are very low. In my practice, I found that half the resultant non-unions of collarbone fractures I treated were painless, and often these results were acceptable to the patient even though complete healing never occurred. Some folks with smaller frames, both men and women, may object to a deformity of the clavicle, and for that reason, primary surgery may be appropriate.

Sternoclavicular Arthritis

The sternoclavicular joint is where the medial (inner) end of the collarbone joins the upper outer portion of the sternum. Sternoclavicular arthritis can occur at that point, but it's not common. If it does occur, conservative management often helps, but in rare instances, surgery may be needed to remove a small portion of the medial clavicle to stop the arthritic changes from rubbing on each other and causing pain or discomfort.

Sternoclavicular Dislocation

A sternoclavicular dislocation is, in theory, a subluxation or partial dislocation. In most instances the medial end of the collarbone never completely separates from the sternum. Mind you, complete dislocations do occur, but they are few and far between. Such a dislocation, like those of the shoulder, can occur either *anteriorly* or *posteriorly*—out of the front of the joint or out of the back, respectively.

A chronic anterior dislocation, meaning it has been present for quite a while, will be quite obvious on physical exam, and even though it is unsightly, if it doesn't cause symptoms, this type of chronic subluxation can be left alone.

In the case of an acute anterior dislocation, the swelling may make diagnosis difficult. If it is recognized, an acute dislocation can be left alone to be dealt with later, or it can be treated by reduction, followed by pinning to hold the reduction in place while ligaments and scar tissue heal around it.

Posterior dislocations are less common than the anterior type and also more difficult to diagnose. If the collarbone's medial end is sufficiently displaced posteriorly, it can compress vital organs (e.g., the major arteries and veins behind the joint). A posterior dislocation is also much more difficult to reduce than the anterior variety. Hyper-extending both of the patient's shoulders over a bolster placed in line with the upper thoracic spine (the mid-portion of the upper back) will sometimes let the collarbone slip back into place, but if it fails to remain there, surgery may be necessary to reduce the dislocation and pin the components in place.

Sterno-costochondritis

Sterno-costochondritis [STERN-o-COS-to-kon-DRY-tis] is a long name for inflammation of the joints that connect the ribs to the sternum. (*Sterno-* refers to the sternum, *costo-* to the ribs, and *chondr-* to the cartilage that lines the bone ends.) In my practice, patients with sterno-costochondritis were almost always young adult females, and the joints involved were the second, third, fourth, and fifth rib attachments, several joints often symptomatic at once.

With sterno-costochondritis, patients will complain mainly of chest pain, often persistent but occasionally intermittent. Any time someone complains of chest pain regardless of their age, the doctor will carry out a careful investigation to rule out disorders of the heart, stomach, and esophagus. I was surprised to learn that, until they consulted me, many of my patients had never had another physician examine them and actually press on the offending joint or joints to confirm the diagnosis.

Sterno-costochondritis is another condition for which conservative treatment is appropriate and the only treatment necessary. Injections of cortisone and local anesthetic usually help alleviate the complaints, but I found that a series of injections was almost always necessary for full relief. I believe that this process is also "self limiting" although, again, it might take quite a period of time to subside.

CHAPTER 6
UPPER ARM BONE (HUMERUS)

Radial Nerve Palsy

Radial nerve palsy is a common complaint associated with the humerus, the arm bone that runs from the shoulder to the elbow. The arm is served by multiple nerves originating from the spinal cord. These nerves travel down the arm to the hand and activate muscles and give sensation to the arm. These nerves from the spinal cord first form the *brachial plexus* [BRAY-key-al PLECK-sus], a conglomeration of nerves coursing from multiple levels of the spinal cord to behind the collarbone and extending into the armpit.

The *radial nerve* originates above the armpit and behind the collarbone, passes into the upper arm, and follows a groove in the middle of the humerus bone. In this area, it is quite superficial, and prolonged pressure on this nerve will cause a radial nerve palsy, an inability to lift one's fingers and hand at the wrist, with numbness and tingling over the back of the hand. This disorder is sometimes called "Saturday night palsy" because it occurs in heavy drinkers who pass out with their upper arm pressed against a chair or a table's edge and remain in that position for a long time. I have also seen it in someone using crutches that were too long and pressed on the radial nerve in the armpit. Such pressure can make the nerve stop functioning and cause a *wrist drop*, a condition in which the wrist flops and the fingers contract into a curled position. The same nerve supplies sensation to the back of the hand, which may also lose feeling.

With relief from the causative pressure, the radial nerve palsy will usually disappear over time, but if the pressure continues for a long period without relief, the lost function may never return, and a surgical procedure to transfer other muscles to function for those affected may be necessary. At surgery, muscles not controlled by this specific nerve are transferred to restore the ability to elevate or lift the wrist and fingers upward or backward (*dorsiflexion*). This intricate, specialized surgery should be performed only by surgeons well experienced in operating on the hand and arm. The operation reroutes these muscles and their tendons to the point of insertion of the affected muscles and tendons. After the surgery, rehabilitation will be necessary to educate the new muscles to perform the functions of the old ones.

Fractures of the humerus can stretch, or even tear, the radial nerve. Anyone with a fracture of the humerus must be examined immediately to determine and document whether the nerve has been injured. Fortunately, many patients will recover from these nerve injuries without surgical intervention.

CHAPTER 7
THE ELBOW

Tennis Elbow

The medical term for tennis elbow, *lateral epicondylitis* [eppie-kon-dil-LIGHT-tis], is a misnomer as it gives the impression that inflammation (*itis*) exists in the *lateral epicondyle* [eppie-KON-dial], the outside tip of the humerus at the elbow. While there may be changes in this area, I and many other orthopaedists believe that the focus of the problem lies in the short tendon origin of one of the muscles that extends the wrist, the *extensor carpi radialis brevis* [ex-TEN-sor car-PEE ray-dee-AL-is BREV-is], or ECRB for short.

Most of my patients with this diagnosis never played tennis or had a history of repetitive sports-related elbow injuries, which led me to theorize that the blood supply at the ECRB tendon's attachment to bone, like the rotator cuff's attachment to the humerus, was probably inadequate, reduced, or absent for some unknown reason. Over time, single or repetitive stresses or simply a lack of sufficient blood will cause inflammation and partial fragmentation or internal tearing of the tendon. The body's response creates scar tissue between the tendon's undersurface and the ligaments and joint capsule of the elbow. The tendon is then bound down so that it becomes adherent to the joint capsule, and it can no longer glide smoothly over the area. Use of the ECRB muscle, in an effort to extend the wrist, then stretches the capsular ligaments, causing pain to radiate from the outside of the elbow to the upper forearm along with acute pain during certain other motions.

Morning stiffness and pain in the elbow are the classic symptoms of tennis elbow, and if the elbow remains at rest for too long, the stiffness can be very annoying and painful with the inability to straighten the elbow for a short period of time. In this condition, like many others, conservative treatment is indicated at first, including anti-inflammatory medications, wet heat, and physical therapy with ultrasound, massage, and electrical stimulation. A compressive band-like brace around the ERCB muscle belly just below the elbow may also help to dissipate pressure on the tendon.

Tennis elbow is one condition in which injections of a refined steroid may be painful and, if not placed in the correct area, may not help at all. In my practice, for this specific injection, I filled a syringe with a fluid mixture of a local anesthetic and a steroid and inserted a small, short 25-gauge needle in the center of the tendon's most tender spot, hoping that hydraulic pressure produced as I injected would separate the tendon from the joint capsule. At times, both the patient and I felt a pop—a good sign—but it didn't always occur. Multiple injections may well be needed over time. This condition will usually subside, but it may take two years. Recurrence of symptoms is relatively common because the initial scar tissue still remains even though there are no symptoms.

In my judgment, surgery is indicated only when the dysfunctional elbow has greatly limited the patient's activities. I once diagnosed tennis elbow in an avid golfer who had an important golf tournament in six weeks. When he said he absolutely needed to healthy by then, I told him it couldn't happen unless I operated immediately. I then described an operation to him that I had never done but had thought through based upon the mechanism of the process outlined above, and he agreed to be the first to undergo the procedure.

The surgery was performed under local anesthesia, so he was awake and able to answer my questions. I was able to locate and remove scar tissue that caused the tendon to adhere to the joint capsule, temporarily placing a rubber material between the structures to prevent a recurrence of adhesion in the immediate postoperative period. The patient was then instructed to move his wrist and fingers up and down as much as possible during the next forty-eight hours. Two days later, I removed the rubber strip, closed its small incision, and told him to continue moving his wrist and fingers as much as possible. He recovered in time to play in the tournament without pain.

I never immobilized these elbow. My results with this approach were most satisfactory to both me and my patients, and in only a few cases did I have to operate again.[12] I am still grateful to that first patient who had enough faith in me to let me perform an operation I had never done but had thoroughly planned in my mind purely on the basis of what I thought was the pathology present with the tennis elbow condition. It was patients like this fellow who made my career so satisfying.

Olecranon Bursitis

Up to this point, the only arm bone we've discussed is the humerus, which connects the shoulder and the elbow. The forearm has two more important bones, the *radius* and the *ulna*, which run parallel to on another between the elbow and the wrist.

A portion of the ulna, the most prominent part of the back of your elbow, is called the *olecranon* [oh-LECK-rah-non] *process*. This part of the ulna forms the cup-shaped part of the elbow into which the end of the humerus fits. Just under the skin and subcutaneous tissue, the olecranon is separated from them only by a bursa. This bursa is easily irritated, easily injured, and can swell. It can also become inflamed, infected by bacteria, or swell as a result of gout.

The Elbow

The most common disorder affecting this area is a relatively chronic yet benign condition known as *olecranon bursitis*. Most of the time, while we have no explanation for the condition, trauma, or repetitive irritation are the most likely causes. Acute and chronic gout or rheumatoid arthritis can also produce this bursitis. In these cases, the bursa swells and the membranous lining releases fluid that accumulates in a loose sac over the tip of the tip of the elbow. This presents as a small floppy balloon on the tip of the elbow filled with fluid. Often, the patient does not even realize it exists.

In the absence of pain or signs of infection or drainage, no treatment is necessary. At other times, however, if the fluid continues to fill the sac until it becomes tense and bulges, the skin over the sac may thin out. Without any drainage or tense distention of the sac, treatment can be delayed, but if a pinpoint drainage site appears, prompt treatment is necessary to prevent infection from entering the sac.

Removing the fluid from this tight sac and injecting refined steroids into it will temporarily relieve the pressure, but the fluid may accumulate again. In that case, surgery to remove the entire sac is the only successful treatment. This surgery is usually performed on an outpatient basis, with complete healing expected within four weeks. Afterward, the body will regenerate another bursa.

In a milder form of this condition, the bursa thickens and adheres to the olecranon in one small area carrying with it some subcutaneous tissue, which causes sharp needlelike pains any time one leans on the elbow and puts pressure on the thickened tissue. In these cases, when doctor presses over the area, he may feel the thickened tissue flip under his finger sometimes reproducing the pain. Folks who have such a bothersome condition generally learn to avoid leaning on that area of the elbow, and over time, the problem areas usually loosen up and cause no more discomfort. If not, an occasional injection may loosen the scarred tissue and diminish symptoms.

Medial Epicondylitis

Earlier, I mentioned lateral epicondylitis, referring to irritation of the outside tip of the elbow bone. *Medial epicondylitis* is much less common, typified by similar pain on the medial or inner aspect of the humerus at the elbow. Examination will reveal tenderness over the short tendon origin of the forearm's flexor muscles on this prominent tip. Medial epicondylitis usually crops up in youngsters who play baseball, especially pitchers. Considered a result of overuse, it can heal if the patient rests the arm and avoids throwing for a time. Adults can also have the condition with or without a history of throwing.

In this condition, the tendon in the area is degenerating more than being inflamed, making *tendinosis* a more accurate term for it. Conservative treatment, circular upper arm bands, and injections usually do the trick, but a few patients may need surgery. During the operation, the surgeon excises a small area of degeneration, scrapes the tendon's attachment site down to bleeding bone, and closes the muscle lining. In this case, like others we've discussed, bleeding from the bone sets up a blood clot that eventually scars, allowing new blood vessels to invade and heal the area.

Osteochondritis Dissecans (OCD)

Osteochondritis dissecans [os-tea-o-chon-DRY-tis dis-SEC-cans] is definitely a challenging term to say. Breaking down the term can help with both pronunciation and grasping its meaning. *Osteo-* refers to bone, and *chondr-* refers to the cartilage lining of the bone in joints. The word *dissecans* has the same Latin root as the verb *dissect*, meaning "to divide into parts."

So *osteochondritis dissecans* tells us there is inflammation and fragmentation of bone and cartilage in a joint that has become partially loose.

Whether the condition is developmental or caused by injury is still up in the air. We know that, for some reason, on the humeral side of the elbow joint, its lateral part or *capitellum* (cap-it-TELL-um) is the area of involvement. The blood supply to this part of the bone just under the joint's cartilage covering loses it blood supply and dies. Reactive inflammation occurs, followed by *avascular necrosis*, which means that the lack of blood vessels leads to bone death. The dead bone tissue then breaks into fragments that loosen under the intact cartilage covering. Remember, the joint cartilage is nourished by the fluid inside the joint and, unlike bone, needs no blood supply.

Continued stress to the elbow will separate the bone fragment from the rest of the humerus with its cartilage covering. The bone piece may be loose while cartilage remains entirely intact, leading eventually to a partially detached piece of bone and cartilage. This may loosen eventually, dropping away from bone to form a loose body in the elbow.

In my practice, I usually saw this condition in girls from ages ten to fourteen, many of them participants in gymnastics. With boys, it was teenage baseball pitchers who subjected their elbows to stress from overuse.

Treatment will depend on the condition of the bone or cartilage fragmentation. If a conservative course of rest, anti-inflammatory medications, and heat fails, surgery may be needed. Several methods can be used: reestablishing the blood supply to the involved area of bone, drilling the bone, replacing the bony fragment in its base, or removing the loose fragment from the joint. After surgery, most aspiring gymnasts with osteochondritis dissecans are unlikely to have an elbow that can withstand the rigors of their sport.

A disorder similar to OCD—*Panner's disease*—occurs acutely in youngsters, usually under the age of ten. X-rays will show only fragmentation of the capitellum bone itself on the outside section of the humerus of the elbow joint. In this case, the fragments never loosen, or is there usually any residual deformity or pain.

Triceps Tendinitis, Tendinosis, or Rupture

The *triceps* is the muscle on the back of the upper arm responsible for extending the elbow or straightening it. This muscle, too, has an associated tendon, and this tendon can become inflamed, deteriorate, or rupture. Any of these disorders can come about from overuse although we know of no specific injury or action that causes them.

The triceps tendon attaches to and envelops the olecranon process of the elbow. When this tendon is affected, pain will be felt over the tendon itself just before its attachment to bone, with tenderness to touch. Conservative treatment is usually helpful, but the tendon can also degenerate and weaken, even to the point of rupture. This is not uncommon in football players, especially offensive linemen who must flex their elbows to block with their hands in front of them, putting the triceps under tremendous stress during each offensive play. Without surgery to repair this tendon rupture, a permanent weakness of the triceps muscle will be the result.

Biceps Tendon Tendinitis, Tendinosis, or Rupture

In an earlier chapter, we discussed the biceps, the two-headed muscle on the front of the upper arm. It attaches at its lower end (the elbow) to the upper portion of the radius, one of the two forearm bones. The upper, concave, rounded end of the radius forms another part of the elbow. Most folks believe the only function of the biceps is flexing the elbow. While it does help with that function, its main job is to *supinate* [SOUP-in-nate] the forearm—to turn the forearm and palm upward. The radius rotates around the ulna, which does not move but acts as a post for the radius to swing on like a gate.

As with any tendon, the biceps tendon can deteriorate (tendinosis once again), fragment, and rupture. Pain arising from the biceps tendon will present in the front of the elbow at its crease, increasing with supination of the forearm against resistance as when a right-handed person turns a tight screw clockwise. Many weightlifters who perform too many biceps curls will suffer this condition. If the biceps tendon ruptures, surgery is not inevitable, but for active young people, it is usually is advised.

Ulnar Neuritis or Neuropathy

The *ulnar nerve* is the classic "funny bone" nerve situated in the *cubital tunnel*, a groove on the side of the elbow next to the body, just behind the bony prominence or medial epicondyle (Fig. 27). At one time or another, you may have whacked your elbow against something, causing a momentary sensation of pins and needles in your hand, and you were told you'd hit your funny bone. It's really not funny and can be quite disabling for a few seconds. Pushing and sliding a finger around in this groove may also pinch this nerve, causing numbness and tingling over the area supplied by that nerve—the little finger and its side of the ring finger next to it.

Occasionally, folks complain of similar symptoms but with no history of trauma or repetitive elbow motions. We say they have *idiopathic neuritis* (nerve inflammation of no known cause). If the inflammation persists, muscles supplied by the ulnar nerve—the muscle between base of the thumb and the base of the second finger, which contracts when pinching, and the muscle in the palm on the little finger side—can atrophy or become smaller. We then say they have *ulnar neuropathy*, meaning there is something wrong with the ulnar nerve that's causing objective or visual evidence of nerve involvement.

Folks may also describe a locking or catching sensation around the ulnar nerve's groove, also associated with the numbness and tingling. In these cases, the covering on the ulnar nerve's groove has loosened so that with certain elbow motions, the nerve will move in and out of the groove, a partial dislocation known as *ulnar nerve subluxation*.

If conservative methods of treatment fail, the only remedy is surgery to transplant the nerve so that it's in front of the groove. Usually highly successful, the surgery is followed by a short period of immobilization of the elbow; active-motion exercises instituted later.

A much less common form of compression of the ulnar nerve causing the same symptoms in the hand can occur in another groove at the wrist known as *Guyon's canal*. The doctor must determine whether the nerve is compressed in this area or in the cubital groove before undertaking any form of treatment.

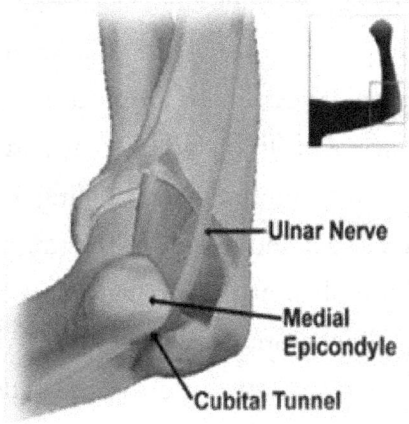

Fig. 27: Medial, inside, view of the left elbow.
Cubital tunnel housing the ulnar nerve.
From the University of Florida Neurosurgery Department

CHAPTER 8
THE WRIST

What an interesting joint! It *seems* simple enough. The hand goes up and down in actions based at the end of the forearm, right? Not exactly. Did you know that there are ten bones that make up the wrist joint?

The bones at the end of the forearm—the radius and the ulna—make up one side of the wrist joint, while four others make up the other side, along with four other intimately attached bones, the *carpal bones.* Granted, the major motion of the wrist occurs between six bones, but the four others must be considered (Fig. 28).

In medical school, we had to memorize the names of these eight carpal bones, along with much more memorization for other body parts. To keep these and others in mind, many of us relied on phrases built around the first letter of each bone's name known as a mnemonic (memory trick). Everyone knew "*Never Loosen Tilly's Pants. Mother Might Come Home*" for the carpal bones, the first letter of each word being the first letter of one of the carpal bones: n*avicular (scaphoid),* l*unate,* t*riquetrum, greater* m*ultangular (trapezium), lesser* m*ultangular (trapezoid),* c*apitate,* and h*amate.* Rather than learning by rote, this gave us a much easier way to memorize lists of terms.

Another mnemonic helped recall the twelve cranial nerves: "*On Old Olympus' Towering Tops, A Finn And German Viewed Some Hops.*" I invented others that were less coherent and, I must admit, a little crude, if not downright gross, but they helped many of us through medical school and specialty training. One thing for sure, we never forgot them while studying for our exams.

But I digress. Let's return to the wrist. We are able to rotate our forearm because of the ability of the radius to rotate around the ulna almost 180 degrees. Although not really a motion of the wrist, in combination with motions of the wrist and our opposable thumb, it enables us to perform intricate maneuvers in many positions. Using certain combinations of muscles, the wrist can also tilt sideways, right and left. For example, when we hold the right palm upward facing ourselves and tilt the wrist to the left, we call that *ulnar deviation* as the hand tilts to the ulnar bone side of the wrist. Tilting to the right, toward the radius side is called *radial deviation.*

Downward motion of the wrist, termed *volar* (toward the palm) *flexion,* is performed by the flexor muscles (the muscles in front of the forearm), while upward motion, or *dorsiflexion* [DOR-see-flex-shun] of the wrist, uses the muscles in back of the forearm (the extensor muscles).

Now you see why the wrist motion is much more than up and down. It can be quite a complicated joint.

The Wrist

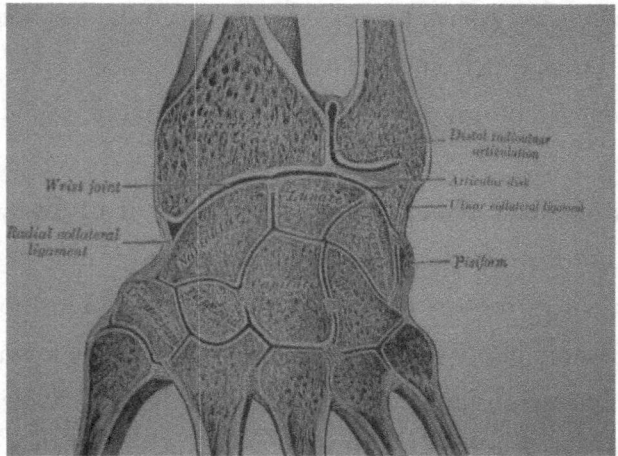

Fig. 28: The carpal bones of a left wrist (8): radius bone (upper left) and ulna bone (upper right). Hand bones: the metacarpals (5) are at the bottom, the thumb being on the left.
Gray's Anatomy, 1966

Sprained Wrist

You may recall that in an earlier chapter, I differentiated between the terms *strain* and *sprain*. Here we're talking about sprains, injury to ligaments. The wrist is susceptible to many injuries, most of them from extreme backward bending (hyperextension) or extreme forward bending (hyperflexion). Because the wrist contains so many ligaments, a combination of ligamentous injuries can occur all at once. The typical treatment for a sprained wrist is ice for the first twenty-four to forty-eight hours, followed by wet heat, rest, and immobilization. A sprained wrist can take quite a while to heal.

Many folks have asked me about the use of ice and heat. After using ice for the first few days to reduce swelling and minimize bleeding, it's appropriate to change over to wet heat in the form of a hot towel or a tub of warm water that increases the blood supply and dilates blood vessels to support the body's healing response.

Some serious injuries can masquerade as sprains. These include fracture of the scaphoid or navicular bone (one of the carpal bones) and disruption of the *scapho-lunate ligament* (the ligament between the scaphoid and lunate bones of the wrist). Pain from these two injuries is similar to that of a sprained wrist, but their symptoms persist much longer than one would expect for a simple sprain.

Fractures of the scaphoid bone may be difficult to diagnose. Regular X-rays may not identify the break in the bone, and it may be necessary to take an X-ray with the wrist tilting to the ulna side. This position better aligns the scaphoid bone with the X-ray beam so that the fracture is visible. Even so, the fracture may not appear at first, but the same X-rays taken three to four days later may reveal it. If the doctor suspects such a fracture, the wrist should be immobilized until the diagnosis is made or ruled out. The reason is that this bone has a less than ample blood supply, and if a fracture disrupts what blood supply there is, a nonunion of the fracture may occur. Long term immobilization of the scaphoid bone break is crucial to allow it to heal, six weeks being the minimal time. If, on the other hand, the fracture is displaced, surgery may be the treatment of choice.

Special X-rays may also be needed to diagnose disruptions of the ligament between the lunate and scaphoid bones, a *scapho-lunate disassociation*. First, a regular X-ray should be made of the wrist, followed by the same view with the patient making and holding a tightly clenched fist. If the ligament is torn, forced clenching of the wrist will produce an intra-articular (inside the joint) pressure and open the space between the two bones produced by the rupture. MRI examination or, in special cases, *arthrography* (injecting a contrast fluid under X-ray control into a joint) may be needed to identify this ligamentous injury.

Another disorder of the wrist that can be quite incapacitating and difficult to diagnose is an injury to the *triangular cartilage* or *articular disc*, a disc or meniscus-like structure found in the wrist joint at the end of the ulna. Pain from this injury will be felt on the end of the ulna at the wrist, increasing with forced tilting to the ulna side, ulnar deviation. An arthrogram or MRI may be needed to make this diagnosis, or arthroscopic surgery may needed for both diagnosis and treatment.

Overall, these sprain-like conditions, especially scaphoid fractures, carpal ligaments, or meniscal injuries, are rather difficult to treat and should be evaluated by an orthopaedic surgeon.

Ganglion Cyst

Probably the most common wrist complaint orthopaedists see is a *ganglion cyst*, a ballooning of the lining of the wrist joint. The wrist, like many other joints, has areas of ligamentous weakness. One such area exists on the back, or dorsal side, of the wrist. Synovial fluid slowly accumulates here from the joint, and with pressures from within the joint, the fluid oozes into a bulging sac or pouch. At some point, a ball or check valve lets fluid in but not out of the joint, and water is eventually absorbed from this fluid, leaving a clear jellylike material. What the patient and the doctor then see is a lump on the back of the wrist (Fig. 29).

Where does its name come from? Ordinarily, a ganglion is an enlargement of a nerve, and I suspect the word was applied to these cysts many years ago because of their bulbous or ballooning character. In the old days, folks called these cysts "Bible tumors" because they would attempt popping the cysts by smashing them with a Bible or another heavy book.

Most of the time, a ganglion cyst causes little pain. In my practice, if it wasn't painful and did not interfere with wrist motion, I always let time take its course to see if it would disappear on its own. If the cyst was painful, removing fluid from it by means of a needle sometimes helped, but in many cases either the needle wasn't large enough to remove the gelatinous fluid or the fluid recurred. If these cysts are *loculated*, separated into different compartments, needling may not help.

About 80 percent of the time, a ganglion cyst will appear on the back of the wrist and about 20 percent on the front or volar side. Cysts on the volar aspect are usually nearer the base of the thumb and can sometimes wrap around an artery, making surgical removal more tedious.

Even with surgery to remove the cyst, there is a chance of recurrence, especially if the joint capsule from which the cyst originates is not removed. I always tried to avoid excising these unless pain was a deciding factor. Just because a ganglion cyst exists and may enlarge is not reason enough to operate on it. Some thin young women may not agree with me, preferring a scar to the lump.

I suspect that many people with ganglion cysts see an orthopaedist before the cyst has become a visible bump, so neither patient nor doctor realizes it's there. Many folks describe a mild to moderate intermittent pain on the back of the wrist, with no history of injury and no evidence of deformity. Examination may not reveal any tenderness, but when asked, most patients can pinpoint the pain at the place where 80 percent of all ganglion cysts eventually appear. I think they're probably describing the beginnings of a ganglion cyst where the dorsal ligaments of the wrist bulge under pressure from the joint. When the cyst actually appears, many of these folks get relief from their symptoms since the tension in the ligaments has been relieved.

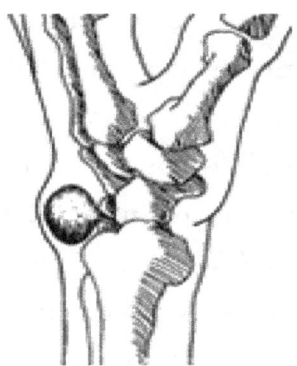

Fig. 29: Dorsal ganglion cyst diagram.
www.deansmithmd.com

Carpal Tunnel Syndrome

The carpal bones form a canal or *U* shape on the palm side of the wrist. This canal is covered by a thick ligament, not unlike the groove of the biceps tendon in the shoulder but much larger and thicker, and rather than a single tendon running through the tunnel, the carpal tunnel accommodates eight tendons and one nerve. In such a tight space, any irritation or inflammation of the tendons or lining will put pressure on this median nerve (Fig 30). Because the median nerve supplies sensation to the palm side of the thumb, the index finger, middle finger, and the middle finger side of the ring finger, pressure on the nerve will cause numbness in these fingers, a condition we call *carpal tunnel syndrome* or *CTS*. No disorder of the median nerve ever causes symptoms in the little finger, however.

If pressure on the nerve continues for long enough, the big muscle on the palm side of the thumb can become smaller, atrophy. The symptoms of carpal tunnel syndrome are most often noticed at night, the reason being that during the day, the hand is generally in constant motion, keeping the swelling down and reducing pressure on the nerve, but at night, with less movement of the hand, there will be more swelling about the tendons and consequently more pressure on the nerve.

Initial treatment for carpal tunnel syndrome is the usual range of conservative measures along with night splints and injections of refined steroid into the tunnel or ligament. If conservative treatment fails, the next step is either open or arthroscopic surgery to relieve pressure in the tunnel by cutting the *transverse carpal ligament* (Fig. 30). I always performed the open procedure as the arthroscopic procedure for CTS was just coming into its own when I retired. Although some surgeons immobilize the wrist for a short period after the surgery, I never did, encouraging my patients to move the hand immediately after the operation. Most folks had immediate relief of the pain and numbness, and most were doing their usual activities two to three weeks after the operation. In most cases, the results of this operation are excellent.

Because many people believe that a repetitive action in a person's job description causes carpal tunnel syndrome, the disorder often qualifies the sufferer for workmen's compensation benefits. I have always disagreed as I saw far more patients whose affliction was unrelated to any job. The majority of my patients who had CTS were female, so while I have no definitive proof of the connection, hormonal changes might conceivably play a role in the disorder.

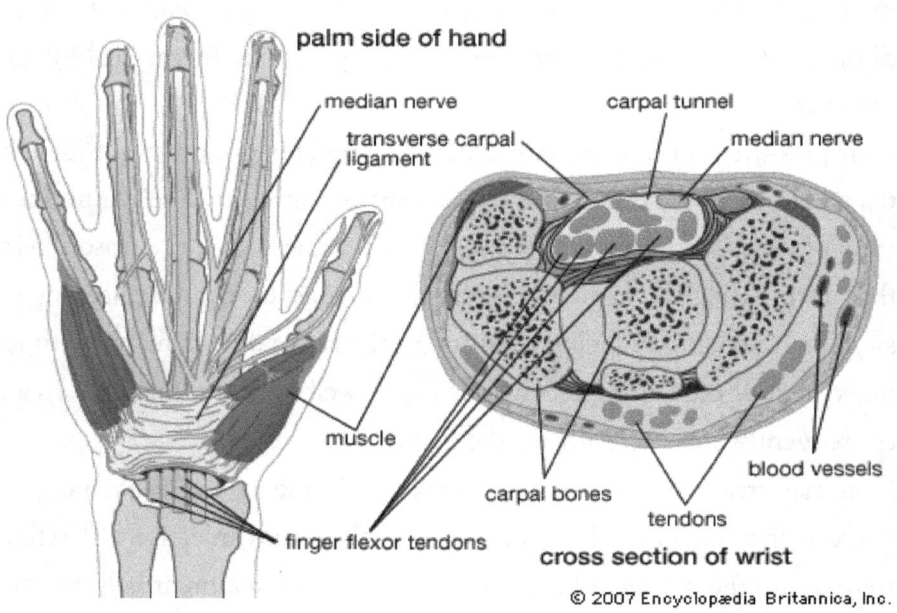

Fig. 30: The carpal tunnel; cross section on right.
Note the transverse carpal ligament .
Notice the number of tendons with the median nerve .
And note that the small finger (diagram on left) has no nerve supply from the median nerve.
Encyclopedia Britannica 2007

CHAPTER 9
THE HAND

De Quervain's Disease

This disorder, named after the doctor who first described it, is otherwise known as *stenosing tenosynovitis of the abductor pollicis longus and the extensor policis brevis.* This long name, which means inflammation of the area around two specific tendons, is quite a mouthful for a small disease process. No wonder physicians put proper names to some conditions. I guess it's for the sake of other tongue-tied physicians.

De Quervain's disease affects the two tendons that lift the thumb. Folks with this condition feel pain over the radius side of the wrist below the thumb, especially in lifting the thumb away from the hand. If the process is present, deviating the wrist toward the ulna forcibly will stretch these tendons and reproduce the pain of De Quervain's disease (Fig. 31)

If you feel around this area, you should find a soft area on the side of your wrist. Now move back ever so slightly to a prominence just before this soft indentation. This is the spot where these two tendons run through a tunnel. Yes, another tunnel! In fact, these tendons occupy and glide through several little tunnels at this point.

Inflammation causes pain that often radiates to the base of the thumb. Medications and injections usually help, surgery being necessary only if other treatments fail. Surgical release of the tunnels, in an outpatient procedure under local anesthesia, will ease pressure on the tendons, usually relieving all the pain. This particular operation is quite successful with very few failures.

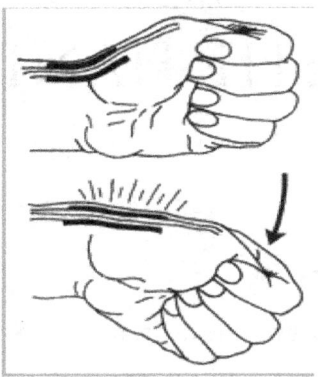

Fig. 31: De Quervain's tenosynovitis
pain pattern elicited with ulnar deviation.
www.deansmithmd.com

Dupuytren's Contracture of the Palm

Dupuytren's contracture, another disorder named for its original describer, is a thickening and contraction of the skin of the palm, usually just off center toward the ring and pinky finger side of the palm. Its cause is also unknown. The condition comes on gradually over a very long time and may never require treatment or surgery even though it can cause enough thickening and contracture of the skin of the palm to pull the ring finger and occasionally the little finger downward. Most folks with a Dupuytren's contracture will often become aware of it only when they can no longer place the palm flat on an even surface. As the contracture begins to pull the finger toward the palm, thickening can be seen at the base of the ring finger (Fig. 32). In more severe cases, the ring finger may bend 90 degrees at the knuckle nearest the palm (the *metacarpophalangeal or MP joint*) with the next joint (the *proximal interphalangeal or PIP joint*) also beginning to flex toward the palm as well. In the most severe cases, the pinky finger will be pulled down in the same manner as the ring finger.

Surgery is indicated only if function is impaired. The operation calls for meticulous dissection and release of the scar tissue, sometimes involving a skin graft.

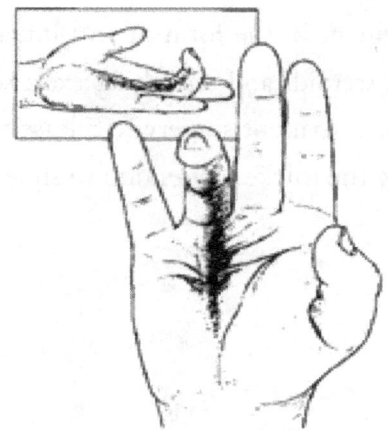

Fig. 32: Duyputren's Contracture pulling the ring finger to the palm.
www.deansmithmd.com

Trigger Finger

Trigger finger, a common disorder of the hand, is a much easier name to remember than the technical term *stenosing tenosynovitis* which means inflammation and thickening of the tendon and its lining. For unknown reasons, the lining of a finger's long flexor tendon becomes inflamed, and the tendon thickens into a localized oval mass just before it enters the base of the finger—still another sheath or tunnel through which the tendon must slide.

If the tendon grows larger than the sheath's entrance, it can't slide easily into it when the finger position changes from flexion to extension (Fig.

33). Initially, the patient may be aware of a popping or snapping sensation, without pain, but as the thickening increases, pain may occur. In some cases, pain at the base of the finger may be the only complaint, the trigger effect coming on later. By *the trigger effect*, I mean a flexed finger that one cannot extend easily and, when applying enough force to straighten it, seems to pop suddenly into extension.

The fingers most commonly subject to this condition are the middle and ring fingers and the thumb although I have seen it in index and pinky fingers as well. Treatment in the form of anti-inflammatory medications, injections of refined steroid, and stretching exercises will usually help. If the problem persists, outpatient surgery to release the tunnel (under local anesthesia) and allow the thickened tendon to slide easily is generally very successful.

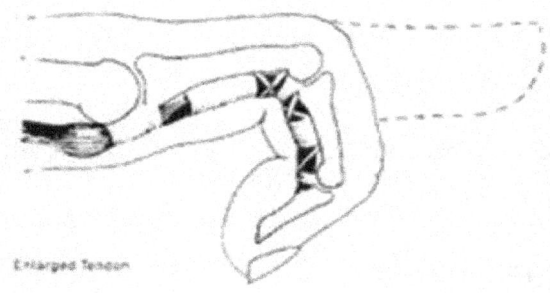

Fig. 33: Trigger finger: notice the oval mass of thickening of the tendon on the left just before it enters the finger. As the finger is straightened, the tendon will snap as it is drawn into and through the tunnel.
www.deansmithmd.com

Carpometacarpal Arthritis of the Thumb

The name of this condition, *carpometacarpal arthritis of the thumb*, tells us two things: there is inflammation in the joint (*arthr-* meaning *joint* and *–itis*) where the long (*metacarpal*) bone at the base of the thumb meets one of the *carpal bones*, the *trapezium* (Fig. 34). This disorder is very common, especially in women forty years of age and older. Pain, usually directly over the joint, with radiation into the thumb, occurs with pinching action as happens when grasping a key to turn it in a lock, turning a tight doorknob, or opening a jar. As the arthritic condition progresses, swelling and deformity may appear, and in the worst cases, the base of the thumb may start to slide outward over a flattened trapezium, moving the rest of thumb's metacarpal bone closer to the index finger.

For some patients, the pain, deformity, or both can be quite debilitating despite conservative management by medication and cortisone injections. When all else fails, surgery can be considered to replace the trapezium with a rolled-up tendon or fusion of the metacarpal bone to the trapezium. Other procedures are available and what works best in your physician's hands is the best course of action. Recuperation after this surgery usually takes at least six weeks and can even take three months, but the relief of pain and restoration of function are quite good and satisfying to the patient.

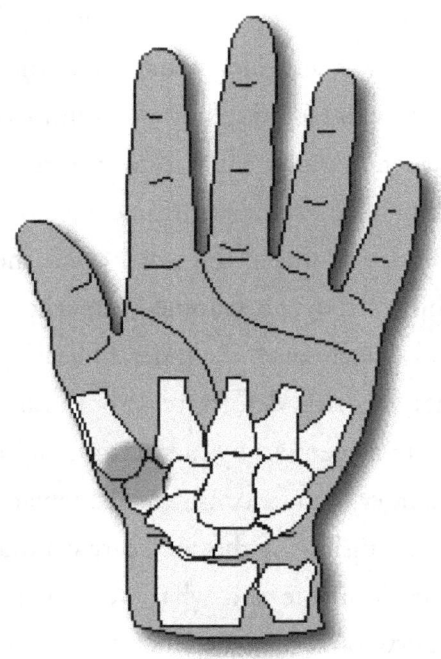

Fig. 34: Location for carpometacarpal arthritis,
gray area at base of the thumb
www.eatonhand.com

Mallet Finger

Mallet finger is the result of a rupture of the extensor tendon that straightens the finger's outermost joint, the *distal interpahalangeal* (DIP) *joint* (Fig. 35). The typical injury happens when one jams one's finger downward, causing the tip of the finger to droop in a deformity that looks like a small hammer, hence the word *mallet*. Sometimes, only the tendon ruptures, but occasionally, a piece of bone is pulled off with it. Appropriate treatment calls for a splint to keep the finger extended for six weeks. If the pulled off piece of bone is large enough, it may cause the DIP joint to become unstable and crooked, necessitating a surgical repair.

Many of these injuries go unrecognized because initial swelling masks the deformity, but as the swelling subsides, the deformity becomes more obvious. Little functional disability accompanies an untreated mallet finger, though a drooping of the joint may be a nuisance for a while until the patient becomes used to it. I know a hand surgeon who has two fingers with such a deformity, neither one ever having been treated. As an internationally known surgeon specializing in the shoulder, arm, and the hand, he gets along very well in spite of these pesky conditions.

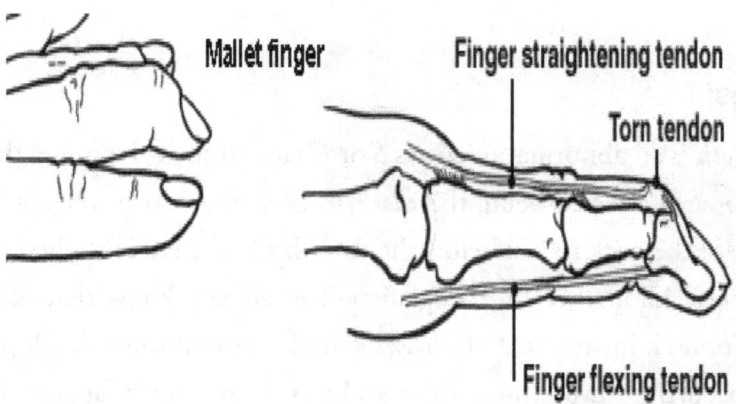

Fig. 35. Mallet finger
www.patient.co.uk/showdoc

CHAPTER 10

THE THORACIC SPINE

Scoliosis

Scoliosis is an abnormal sideways S or C curvature of the spine, the most common area affected being the *thoracic spine*, the part of the spine from the base of the neck to just below the twelfth rib, the last rib. There are two main types: idiopathic and congenital. You already know that *idiopathic* means "of no known cause." *Congenital* indicates that some developmental defect occurring in utero caused a scoliosis to eventually appear. One or multiple vertebrae may fuse together on one side, and as the child grows, the fused area does not mature as quickly, allowing the spine to grow faster on one side and therefore developing a curvature. Most of the cases seen by the orthopaedist in his office are idiopathic. Females definitely outnumber males. We used to see scoliosis mainly at ages ten and up, but with the advent of scoliosis screenings in schools, some cases are seen earlier.

I used a simple method to examine this curvature to get an initial idea of how serious the curve was. I'd have the child stand with her back to me and relax, and I'd feel the upper spine area for the highest spinous process of the thoracic spine. This bony extension of the covering of the back of the vertebra arch can be felt in the middle of the back (Fig. 36). Using my index and middle fingers pressed together, I'd then place this prominence between my fingers and, with a gentle but increased pressure, slide my fingers down the back, keeping each subsequent spinous process between my fingers as I descended. I'd do this three or four times, creating a red blush in the skin over these bumps. Standing back, I could identify a curve by whether the line of red skin was straight or curved. Granted, this is a technique that would not pick up small curvatures, but it did give me something to go on. If there was an obvious curve, an X-ray was taken, and the angle and position of the curve documented. Experience taught me that if the red line was straight, there was usually no curve or only a minimal curve, and no X-ray would be necessary.

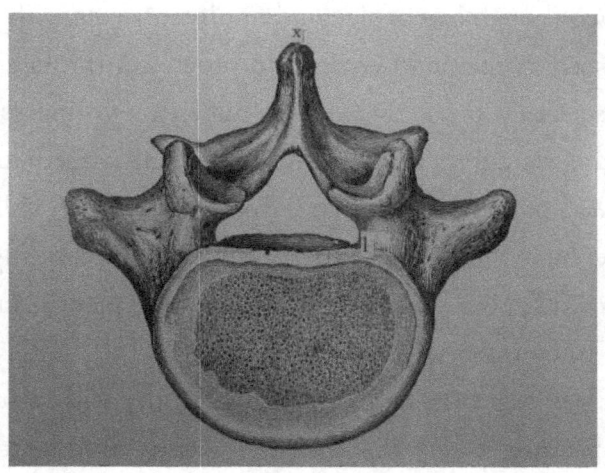

Fig. 36: Cross-section example of a vertebra: note the spinous process (x), the bony prominence at the top. The spinal nerves exit the triangle through grooves on the right and left of the lower edges of the triangle (1- on right).
Gray's Anatomy, 1966

Patients were checked every six months, and if the red lines documented in the chart were considered more prominent than during the last visit, an X-ray would be taken to check the degree of curve. If there was no change, a yearly visit was suggested. I, as well as the parents, was always worried about the radiation that children were subjected to, especially girls, with the developing breast being directly within the X-ray beam. Precautions were always taken: lead breast covers for females and gonadal protective devices for males. The amount of radiation emitted during a scoliosis exam with two views would equal approximately 10 millirads, whereas dental X-rays may emit 1,000 millirads. To put it in perspective, if you stayed in a brick building twenty-four hours a day for a year in New York City, you'd be exposed to 140 millirads. But radiation is radiation, and I tried to use as little as I could, especially in the case of growing children.

Usually, no treatment is necessary for mild scoliosis other than follow-up until the child has finished growing. Curves under ten degrees are sometimes not considered to be true scoliosis, but I prefer to call any curve a scoliosis even though it is benign and not intensifying with age. Scoliosis tends to worsen as the child enters and progresses through puberty and gets taller, especially the early years of puberty. Treatments for scoliosis include bracing for curves from 25–40 degrees and surgery for curves over 40 degrees. Again, treatment depends on a child's age. A child with a 30- or 35-degree curve who is close to finishing her growth might not need any treatment at all, but with a younger child with plenty of time to grow, surgery may be considered.

A case of scoliosis with an increasing deformity will create a *rib hump* on one side because of both the intensifying curve and the rotation of the vertebrae of the spine (Fig. 37). You see, not only does the spine bend with this process, it also rotates the more severe it gets. In this diagram, notice how the spinous processes on the top and the bottom of the curve are in the middle of the back, but in the midsection of the curve, they have rotated off center. This rotation causes the ribs to become more prominent on one side—the rib hump—and in some cases, the lower aspect of the ribs on the other side actually touch the pelvis wing. Fortunately, there are very few severe cases of scoliosis, but it's wise to check your child often. If any concerns arise, see an orthopaedist.

There are no symptoms from scoliosis unless the curves are so severe as

The Thoracic Spine

to restrict motion or breathing. These children have no pain or discomfort and usually have no idea that a curve exists. Parents should be observant and occasionally check their teenagers' backs for more prominent ribs on one side, a shoulder that's higher than the other, a sideways curve to the spine, or a hip that's higher than the other.

There is no need to protect these children from playing any sport or performing any activity unless, of course, they are wearing a brace. Using a brace for treatment does not straighten the curve. It helps to prevent the curvature from worsening.

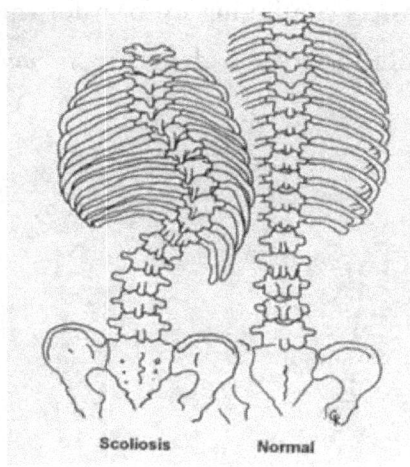

Fig. 37 : Scoliosis diagram: note the C curve on the left and how the ribs on the right side of this diagram bunch up together as a result of curving and rotating forming a rib hump
www.youngwomenshealth.org

Shingles/Herpes Zoster

Anyone who has had chickenpox is at risk for the development of shingles although it occurs most commonly in people over the age of sixty. After one has chickenpox, this virus—*varicella zoster*—lives in the nervous system and never fully disappears from the body. It usually lies *dormant*, hidden away, in the thoracic nerves that lie between the ribs and originate from the thoracic spinal cord, but the virus can affect nerves elsewhere in the body. These thoracic nerves supply the skin with its sensation from the back to the center front of the rib cage. Orthopaedists usually see this disease when it affects the nerves around the thoracic cage because of pain that suddenly appears with no identifiable cause.

The patient may notice the onset of a burning pain and sensitive skin, with the skin sensitivity usually lagging behind the pain. The pain can be severe, necessitating narcotic medications. The sensitive skin area eventually exhibits a rash. Before the rash is visible, it may be difficult to determine the cause of the severe pain. The shingles rash starts as small red blisters, with new blisters continuing to form for three to five days. The blisters follow the thoracic nerves' path or *dermatomal patterns* (Fig. 39).

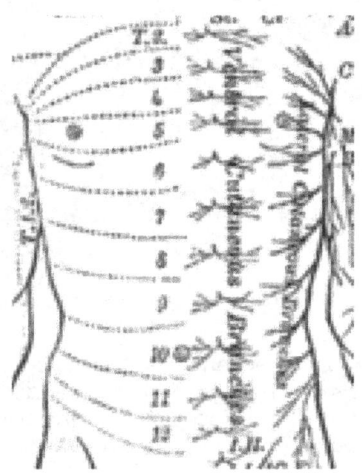

Fig. 39: The levels (dermatomes) of skin supplied by the thoracic nerves
http://en.wikipedia.org/wiki/Dermatomic_area

The rash does not cross the midline of the body. The entire path of the nerve may be involved, or there may be skipped areas. Generally, only one nerve level is involved. In a rare case, more than one nerve can be involved. Eventually, the blisters pop, and the area starts to ooze, finally crusting over and healing. The whole process may take three to four weeks or more. On occasion, the pain will be present and the blisters never appear. The pain of shingles is persistent and continuous and can be debilitating until the process ends.

Shingles is contagious, but chickenpox is usually the disease transmitted. Once they have had chickenpox, people cannot contract the virus from someone else. Once infected by chickenpox, however, people have the potential to develop shingles later in life. Shingles is contagious to people who have not had chickenpox as long as new blisters are forming and old blisters are healing. Once all the blisters are crusted over, the virus can no longer be spread.

There is a vaccine, Zostavax, for shingles. The Center for Disease Control and Prevention (CDC) has recommended the vaccine for everyone over sixty years of age. The vaccine cuts the occurrence of shingles by about 50 percent in adults sixty and over, according to the CDC. For those from sixty to sixty-nine, it is 64 percent effective.

CHAPTER 11
THE THORACOLUMBAR SPINE

The *thoracic spine* is relatively rigid compared with the neck (the *cervical spine*) and the low back (the *lumbar spine*). This is because it is encased in twenty-four ribs, twelve on the right and twelve on the left (Fig. 37). The ribs are also attached to the *sternum*, the chest bone in front that creates a barrel of sorts. This construct houses the lungs and the heart within a protective cage. There are twelve thoracic vertebrae. Since there is minimal motion in all planes in the thoracic spine, very few problems associated with disc degeneration exist here. However, at the interval of the thoracic and the lumbar spine, there is an abrupt transition because of the absence of ribs. Whenever a more rigid structure meets a flexible one, more stresses occur; therefore, at the T12–L1 level, the area between the twelfth thoracic and the first lumbar vertebra, patients often develop pain secondary to arthritic joint changes and degenerative discs.

The symptoms can be described as pain radiating from the midline of the back out to and below the last ribs of the back, often misdiagnosed as kidney problems. In Fig. 40, the T12–L1 level is the area between the last (twelfth) vertebra, with its small rib, and the vertebra below, L1 (lumbar one). This is the area of transition from the green-colored vertebra and the purple ones. The symptoms can be intermittent or constant, rarely severe.

Prolonged sitting may increase the pain. Most patients will report that the pain is centered in a spot just off the midline of the back, either the right or the left. Conservative treatment is usually all that is necessary for this condition.

I mention this condition because it is often not diagnosed initially, and the symptoms may go on for quite some time before it is found to be the cause. X-rays may show some changes in this area, but many times, the changes are minimal and may be overlooked. A bone scan may identify increased uptake of the radioactive material in the facet joints of the vertebra in this area and help identify the problem.

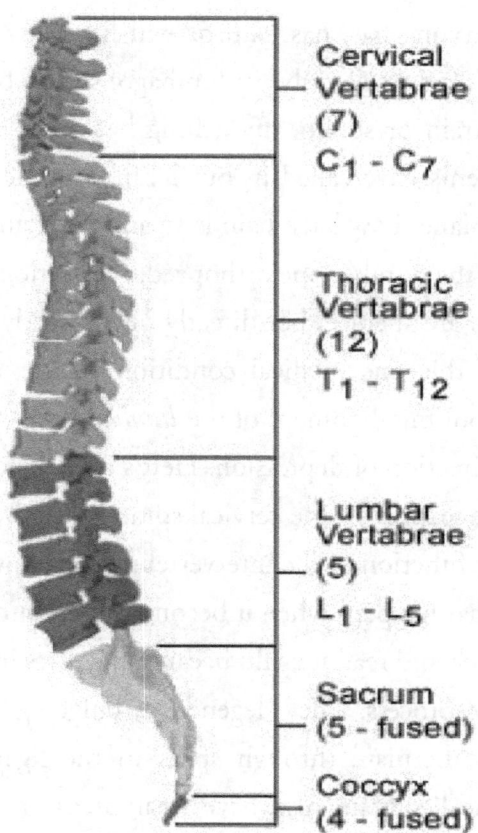

Fig. 40: Spinal column: note the specific sections
www.sci-recovery.org

CHAPTER 12
LUMBO-SACRAL SPINE

Low Back Pain

Just about everyone has, has had, or will have low back pain. Many words have been used to describe it: lumbago, sciatic back pain, sciatica, lumbar muscle strain or sprain, my aching back, etc. I'm sure there are other names patients have called it, but I can't use them here since they border on the profane. Low back pain is so annoying and so disturbing to one's life that it is the number one orthopaedic condition seen in the office. Billions of dollars are spent either directly or indirectly on the treatment or prevention of this one medical condition yearly. The causes of the problem range from misalignment of the *lumbar spine*—the low back—to psychologic misdirection of depression. Here's my take on it.

If you read the section on the cervical spine, you now understand what I believe to be the function of the intervertebral disc, how it works when it is normal, and what happens when it becomes dried out or degenerative. I suggest you go back and read it again because the discs in the lumbar spine undergo the same process. They degenerate, bulge against the ligaments holding them in, herniate through splits in the ligaments, and cause referred pain. The ligaments also have weak areas on the left and right as seen in Fig. 5. When stretched, the pain is often referred to the right or left in the low back and/or the buttock. When referred to the right or left, many people erroneously think muscles are involved and therefore a muscle strain exists. Many patients will only have just low back pain, some will have buttock pain and complain of no low back pain at all, and some will have both.

When a nerve in close proximity to the bulging disc is irritated, pain in the back of the upper thigh, *upper posterior*, can occur with radiation to the back of the knee. Some call this *sciatica*. The reference here is to the sciatic nerve. It is formed by a conglomeration of five major nerves from the fourth lumbar area to the third sacral level. The sciatic nerve travels down the back of the leg where it eventually splits into two nerves behind the knee joint. Because pain is often referred along its anatomic distribution, the word *sciatica* has been used as a diagnosis, but it doesn't necessarily mean that any specific nerve or the whole sciatic nerve is involved.

Most of the motion of the *lumbar spine*, the low back, occurs between the L4 and L5 vertebra (L4-5) as well as the L5 vertebra and the first sacral vertebra, S-1 (L5-S-1) and their disc spaces and respective joints. The rest of the motion occurs from L1-2, L2-3, and L 3-4 disc spaces and their joints. The discs of the lumbar spine will degenerate as I have described, and since most of the motion is centered at L4-5 and L5-S1, more degeneration will occur here than the other levels. S1 is the top of the sacrum, and the sacrum is made up of five vertebrae, but they are all fused together, so there is no motion of these bones on one another (Fig. 40).

When the disc at L4-5 bulges acutely, *acute low back pain*, the patient often is incapacitated and unable to move, tilted to one side, bent over, and unable to straighten up. Usually, when L5-S1 disc bulges, there is no tilting of the spine, but muscle spams will accompany it, keeping the patient from straightening up. The muscles about the spine are in true spasm, protecting the disc from bulging any further and not allowing the patient to move. It can happen anytime: lifting an object, getting in and out of a car, arising from a sitting position, arising from a bent over position, or even in one's sleep. It is not caused by one movement. It is the straw that breaks the camel's back, so to speak. Let me explain.

I have discussed how the disc fragments within their confines eventually are pushed around by forces applied to the disc space by everyday activity. It is my contention that these forces are at play all the time even when one is rolling over in bed, but the most force upon a disc space occurs when we bend over from the waist. It has been estimated that the pressure within the disc space with the torso bent forward at 45 degrees is greater than six hundred pounds per square inch. The reason for such a high pressure is that the *paravertebral muscles*, those muscle situated around the spine, are pulling back as hard as they can so the person doesn't fall forward and thereby compress and increase the pressure within the lumbar disc spaces. Each time this force is applied, the disc material is compressed and moves slightly toward the back, *posteriorly*. It may take quite a number of moves for a loose piece of disc to travel far enough to bulge the ligament and cause symptoms.

Please understand that I am trying to explain the mechanism in layman's terms to convey my thoughts about how disc disease progresses. Let's say, for sake of argument, it takes two hundred times bending at the waist to bulge a disc. If this occurs over a one-month period, pain will occur every month, but the episode may take quite awhile to disappear so the low back pain seemingly persists all the time. However, if those two hundred times could be spread out over a year period, one would have a mild episode that would disappear over time, leaving him pain free. I know this is a simple way to describe the overall mechanics, but stay with me on this.

The ultimate answer would seem to be spreading those bending moments over as long a period as possible. Therefore, in order not to apply abnormal forces to our discs, we all should keep our backs perpendicular or parallel to the ground at all times because these are the positions where the least amount of pressure exists within the disc spaces. Not so easy if you think about it, but that's just what people need to do, *think about it!* Consciously, one should never bend from the waist, and if one must, then he should place his hand or hands on something so the weight of the torso and body are placed on a hand or hands reducing the amount of paravertebral muscle contraction so they don't need to pull as hard and therefore decreasing disc space pressures. When arising from the bent position, everyone should bend their knees enough so their back is again in the perpendicular stance, then let their hands loose and stand straight up. If we are not able to use our hands in the manner described, then all bending should be performed very slowly to avoid sudden or fast motions. This allows the pressure to build up slowly within the space. Of course, there are times when we do not have full control over our bodies, and we must use the lower back incorrectly. We would just have to accept that specific move as one of the two hundred improper uses of our low back.

Did you know that the pressure in disc spaces is higher when sitting than standing upright? Muscles are acting when we are upright thereby dissipating some of the weight from the lower spine, but these muscles mostly relax in the sitting position, allowing the weight of the head, upper extremities, and torso to be applied to the lower back. That is why prolonged sitting increases low back pain. It is imperative to get out of a seated position as often as possible, even if it were just for only a few minutes. But you have to watch the way you get out of a chair or car too!

Check yourself very carefully as you get out of a chair the next time you are in a restaurant or at the kitchen table. Normally, one leans forward approximately 45 degrees, placing the middle of one's torso over his feet. In other words, we move our center of gravity over our feet to stand up. Once in that position, we are in the position I mentioned above, bent from the waist without our hands on anything. We then stand up placing a higher pressure on our disc spaces. How many times do you get out of a sitting position a day? If you get up as I described, then you are using your back incorrectly that many times a day. A little frightening to think about, right?

So how are we supposed to stand up? Place you feet under your chair instead of placing your body over your feet. This places the feet under our center of gravity instead of vice versa. Move your buttocks to the front of the chair, and now you can stand straight up using your thigh muscles without any bending at the waist keeping your back perpendicular to the floor. This is a simple physical principle, but remembering to do so is a most difficult and daunting task. We must educate ourselves constantly until it becomes second nature. Believe me, I know.

I developed low back pain after an acute episode when I was twenty-five years old. It was like my lower back totally seized up on me, and no matter what I did, I couldn't move very well. There was no way I could get out of bed after "pulling a muscle" in my back the night before. I had to crawl on the floor to get around. The episode gradually improved over several days, but I continued to have this type of episode off and on. Through these attacks, I noticed my body was trying to tell me something. I realized that I had to place my feet under me to avoid bending when standing up because the muscle spasms and pain wouldn't let me do otherwise. I had to place my hand or hands on objects to get things off chairs and the floor without adding undue pressure to my back and increasing the pain. If I had the pain, there were only several ways I could move, my back perpendicular or parallel to the floor. If it was imperative to perform these actions with pain, why shouldn't I do them without pain to protect the disc from bulging as well? It seemed obvious that those motions were only allowed while I was in pain, presumably to prevent further consequences, and therefore, if I performed them when I felt normal, shouldn't that help prevent or at least decrease the number of episodes? To me, the answer was yes.

I quickly found that sleeping on my stomach aggravated my back pain because it hyper-extended my spine, adding more pressure to the discs.

Lying in bed with my hips and knees bent or with my knees draped over large pillows would flatten my back and relieve pressure. Lying on my side with my knees curled up did the same. I did not learn these tricks quickly. I didn't have knowledge of the anatomy of the spine at that time, but gradually, I started to incorporate these actions into my daily life until they were second nature. How? It will sound silly, but if you—lying in bed just before falling to sleep—consciously repeat, "I will not sleep on my stomach. If I do, I will wake up and change position," eventually, you will awake on your stomach one night. It is then most important that you change position to your side or on the back with the knees bent. Continuing to do this will educate your body to do so without you consciously repeating the statement.

Do I always use my back properly? Heck, no! But if I can do it during all controlled periods of the day, I reduce my chances of another low back pain episode. In other words, I spread my two hundred wrong moves over a longer period of time. Will this work for everyone? I doubt it, but it should allow most patients a mechanism to control and dissipate the forces on the lumbar spine to help avoid the degenerative discs from being compressed and bulged. It is certainly worth everyone's time and attention to avoid what can be a most unpleasant attack of low back pain.

The initial treatment for acute low back pain is rest, anti-inflammatory medications, and heat. We used to admit these patients with severe episodes to the hospital, but we soon discovered that prolonged rest and immobilization often was counterproductive. The use of mild pain medications and NSAIDs are usually the first line of defense. It may be necessary to use a six-day decreasing course of a cortisone derivative for its anti-inflammatory effect. Gradual reduction of pain should be followed by ambulation. Should the episode not improve, one should seek medical advice, especially if there is pain or numbness and tingling in the leg.

Herniated Lumbar Discs

These herniations are similar to the cervical spine disc herniation. The disc gradually oozes out of its space through the ligament (*chronic herniated disc*) or is suddenly extruded (*acute herniated disc*). The chronic herniation occurs over time usually with the symptoms of the bulging, splitting, or tearing of the ligament, followed by the extrusion of the disc material through the ligament into the area where the nerve is present and/or into the *lateral recess*, the groove/tunnel that the nerve travels in as it exits the vertebral area altogether (Fig. 41). There are multiple variations of herniations: a large piece totally isolated outside the disc space compressing the nerve, *complete rupture or herniation*; partial herniation, *protrusion*, with part of the disc totally out and part still within the space and/or caught in the ligament; the disc has displaced itself by stripping off the ligament from the bone causing the disc to be interposed between the bone and ligament sometimes large enough to compress a nerve; or a combination of these.

The L4-5 disc herniation will compress the L5 nerve causing pain in the buttock and leg pain down to the foot with numbness and tingling over the top of the foot, especially in the skin between the first and second toes. Lifting one's leg straight up while supine will increase the pain and the ability to do so will be severely limited. If enough pressure has occurred to the nerve, weakness of the muscles of the lower leg that lift the foot up—the *dorsi-flexors of the ankle and big toe*—will be involved. This can be tested by trying to walk on one's heels. If there is weakness of these muscles, the foot will settle back to the floor and not remain elevated.

The L5-S1 herniated disc will cause the same type of pain, but the numbness and tingling are usually on the bottom of the foot with eventual weakness of the calf muscles, *plantar flexors of the foot and ankle*, and the decreased ability to walk on one's tiptoes. Straight leg raising will be reduced and painful, and on physical exam, the ankle reflex—obtained by tapping the Achilles tendon—will be reduced or absent

Occasionally, we will see a herniated disc at L3-4. The symptoms will also include leg pain, often not traveling past the knee. The leg pain will tend to be in front of the upper leg, the thigh. Numbness and tingling will occur over the front aspect of the thigh and, eventually, weakness in the thigh muscle, the *quadriceps*, and decreased or absent knee jerk reflex.

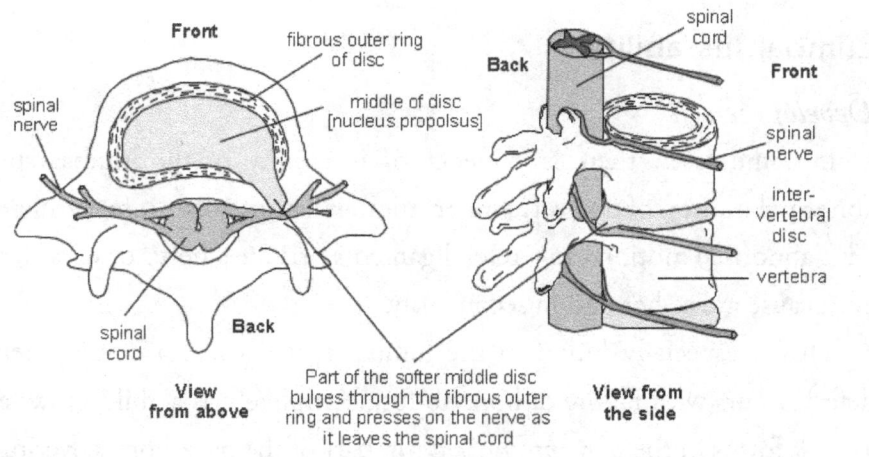

Fig. 41: Diagram of herniated lumbar disc.
Note the nerve compression by the disc fragment.
www.patient.co.uk

Treatment for all of these include anti-inflammatory medication, possibly a course of cortisone, rest, physical therapy, heat, massage, ultrasound, electrical stimulation, and epidural cortisone injections. These injections are given into the spinal canal from outside around the lining of the nerve, the *dura*, hopefully locally reducing the inflammation caused by the herniated disc. A series of these are usually given. With the failure of these modalities, surgery could be considered. Nowadays, microscopic surgical and laser techniques allow the surgeon to approach the disc through small incisions disrupting very little tissue. Some bone covering the back portion of the spinal canal on the side of the herniation is removed, the nerve identified, pulled aside, and the disc material causing the compression is removed.

Any surgeon performing this procedure should explain all the available techniques to the patient, the rehabilitation, the complications, and their success rate. Some herniations do not fit well with the microscopic procedure, and these are usually evident by the MRI.

Lumbar Instability

Developmental

In some cases, there is evidence of instability of the lumbar spine: abnormal motion of one vertebra on another causing discomfort and pain. This abnormal motion can stretch ligaments, irritate a nerve or nerves, and even cause a disc herniation secondarily.

This is especially found in the lumbar spine where a developmental defect occurs with failure of bone to fuse completely as a child grows and a crack forms in the *pars intraarticularis*, part of the back bony covering of the vertebra on either side of the spinous process, *spondylolysis* [SPON-dil-o-LIE-sis]. This can be found on one side or both. When the defects are on both sides, they can lead to small stress fractures or cracks in the vertebrae that can weaken the bones so much that the front part slips away from the back covering and slips on the vertebra below, a condition known as *spondylolithesis* [SPON-dil-o-LITH-thi-sis] (Fig. 42). The more slippage, the more the instability. This usually occurs at either L5-S1 or L4-5.

Conservative measures are the first line of defense, but surgery to correct the slippage and/or fuse the bones in the correct position may be necessary to stabilize the spine. In the old days, fusions were carried out without using any mechanical devices, but techniques to utilize screws and plates have been so perfected that the results are more stable and seemingly better now. Spine surgery of this type is usually not performed by a general orthopedist but one who has had extra training in doing so.

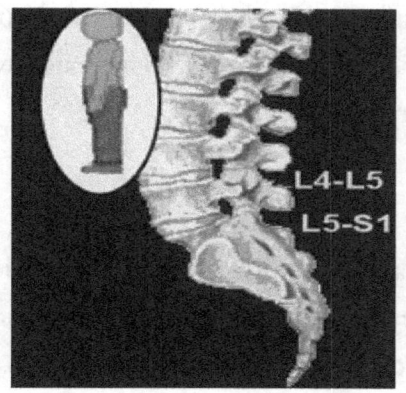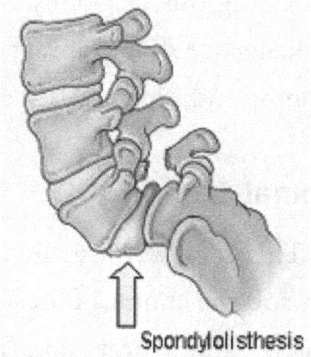

Fig. 42: Normal position of L5 vertebra on S1, left; Slippage or spondylolithesis of L5 on S1, right. www.easyvigour.net.nz Area of original defect (x) www.back.com

Lumbar Instability Secondary to Disc Degeneration

With disc space narrowing, the joints behind the vertebra can become offset thereby developing ligamentous loosening and stretching around them. This can lead to a chronic instability of the two vertebrae involved. The looseness of the joints allows each side to become offset against the other promoting subsequent joint lining inflammation and actual physical irritation of the joint surfaces leading to arthritis and pain. The problem here is the diagnosing which level or levels are involved. This can be very difficult and needs a physician very experienced in dealing with these conditions. A *degenerative spondylolithesis* can occur secondary to this type of loss of disc space. The joints become offset, ligaments loosen, gradual flattening and malformation of the bones forming the joints occurs, and a subsequent sliding of one vertebra on the other can result.

A fusion may be the only treatment left, but what two or three vertebras should be operated? Certain diagnostic modalities will be necessary, including flexion and extension X-ray views, MRI evaluations, and possible local *facet joint* anesthetic injections to reveal the center of instability. Since evaluating this instability is most difficult to completely understand and evaluate, one should always seek the advice of a physician who has extensive training and experience in spinal stability surgery.

Spinal Stenosis

This condition usually comes with aging. As discussed, the disc dries out and the annulus fibrosis strands break up and thin out; the disc space height reduces over time. The joints behind the vertebra—*facet joints*—become offset, rub together, and, eventually, arthritic changes occur. The hyaline cartilage inside these joints eventually disappears, and bone rubs on bone often stretching the ligaments that surround the joints.

As a result, the ligaments pulling on the lining of the bone form spurs, *osteophytes* [OS-teo-fights], that can grow quite large and impinge upon the adjacent nerves and other structures. These arthritic changes and bone spurs in the joints behind the disc spaces, combined with degenerative disc space, collapse as well as infolding and thickening of the ligaments between the bony vertebral arches (*ligamentum flavum*) all lead to narrowing (*stenosis*) of the triangle where the spinal nerves are as well as the grooves and tunnels (*lateral recesses*) where the nerves exit (Fig. 43).

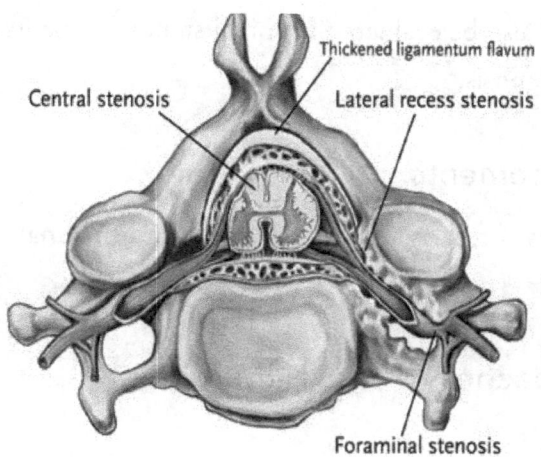

Fig. 43: Spinal Stenosis: Note the compression of the spinal sac and nerves (nerve roots) from the thickened ligaments centrally and vertebral boney growths, osteophytes, on the right
Courtesy of Medtronic Sofamor Danek USA, Inc.

The symptoms of *spinal stenosis* can be low back pain, but mostly buttock and leg pain often without the neurologic deficits that are present with the herniated discs. The pain can be severely debilitating, leading to the inability to walk long distances, stand for long periods, and just perform the activities of daily living. Unfortunately, this condition comes with aging and the presence of an arthritic condition about the joints and disc spaces. I know of no prevention of this process. Some folks are unlucky enough to develop it, whereas others do not.

Conservative management usually is only helpful for short periods of time. When the patient's life style is disturbed enough, surgery to remove part of the back arch covering of the vertebra (the *lamina*) decompress the spinal nerves (*decompressive laminectomy*) and relieve the compressive effects of the stenosis by osteophytes and thickened soft tissue is usually highly successful.

Some patients with vascular disease of their arteries leading to their legs can develop pain and symptoms similar to that of spinal stenosis. Arterial disease should also be evaluated in spinal stenosis patients to be absolutely sure of the diagnosis.

Disc Replacements

This surgery, I feel, is still in its infancy, and the final long term results are not in yet.

New Approaches to Disc Herniations

Nucleoplasty

Nucleoplasty is a minimally invasive procedure developed to treat patients with contained or mildly herniated discs. A special needle is placed into the disc space using X-ray. A wand-like device is then inserted through the needle and into the disc. Heat is transmitted through the device to cauterize and remove the disc material as well as sealing the tract made by the needle. Multiple channels are used, depending on how the amount of disc needed to be removed.

Ozonucleolysis

This procedure injects ozone into the disc space causing shrinkage of the disc thereby reducing its volume and lessening pressure on the nerves.

Intradiscal Electrothermal Therapy (IDET) or Intradiscal Electrothermal Annuloplasty (IDEA)

This thermo-coagulation procedure—heat used to coagulate disc material—is minimally invasive and usually done under local anesthetic. This surgery is generally recommended for patients with contained disc herniations only. The coagulation, in theory, causes the disc material to reform back into the center of the disc space. The surgery is not recommended for ruptured discs or discs out of their confines.

All these procedures are relatively new, and the results are not completely in on any of them. They do seem to have potential especially since they are minimally invasive, and the long-term results will spell out the true effects of the theories behind them.

CHAPTER 13
THE PELVIS AND HIP JOINTS

Sacroiliitis

Sacroiliitis [SAY-kro-il-lee-i-tis] is an inflammatory condition of the *sacroiliac joint or joints*. These joints are formed where the wings of the pelvis connect to both sides of the sacrum or tailbone. Sudden onset of fever, pain and decreased range of motion, limping, and general overall fatigue are symptoms, but many patients often complain about just one or two of these. Overall, I can remember only a few patients who actually had more signs than direct tenderness over the sacroiliac joint that's consistent with this process. A differential diagnosis of infection, rheumatoid arthritis, herniated disc, and possibly ankylosing spondylitis (a chronic, often painful inflammatory arthritis affecting joints in the spine and the sacroiliac joints in men, causing eventual fusion of the spinal vertebrae) must be entertained before finalizing the diagnosis and treatment.

I can recall several cases of pregnant patients who developed symptoms consistent with sacroiliitis secondary to the increased laxity of ligaments present with all pregnancies. The symptoms slowly disappeared after delivery.

Although I never saw such a case, others have identified this condition in patients with severe drug addictions. Chronic or acute infections of this joint can occur due to the introduction of bacteria into the bloodstream by the use of non-sterile needles.

Coccydynia

Coccydynia [kox-sa-DIN-e-a] is truly a pain in one's rear. Not only for the patient but often for the physician who is treating it. Its cause is unknown, and many physicians do not consider it a disease process, considering the patient is depressed, faking the symptoms, or attempting to get attention.

Most of the cases I treated were in women, all of whom definitely had moderate to severe pain over the tip of *the coccyx*, the most distal portion or tip of the sacrum. Normally, there is no redness and no swelling, but there is exquisite tenderness over this movable portion of the coccyx. Anatomically, this area of the coccyx has many muscles and ligaments attached, especially in women where the reproductive organs are supported. This may be an answer as to why women have more problems with this condition than men.

X-rays are not usually helpful but should be taken in order to rule out any infection or tumorous condition. The usual treatments include anti-inflammatory medications, heat, and avoiding pressure on the distal coccyx by use of inflatable rubber doughnut-type devices. Some physicians have used manipulation of the coccyx through the rectum, but I have never heard of a patient responding to this maneuver.

With failure of these treatments, I often used an injection of refined steroid and a local anesthetic. I tried to introduce the needle above the tip of the coccyx and place it under the *periosteum*, the lining of the bone. I believe the pain is a result of a *periostitis* (inflammation of the periosteum, the liming of bones) of the coccyx bone. It makes sense to me that that a repetitive stretching of this periosteum by other structures would eventually create an inflammatory response at the center of the process. The injection can be painful because there is no space to inject; however, once the local anesthetic begins to work, the original pain will subside, giving the patient relief and proof that there is a process present—it's not just in their head. Unfortunately, the response to the injections may not cure the problem, and other injections may be necessary. The symptoms can last for months or years, but at least, physicians can relieve the pain for some periods of time.

Total surgical excision of the coccyx is a last resort, and often, the pain is not relieved with this procedure. The reason, I believe, is that the problem is actually in the ligamentous support structures rather than the bone itself. Excision of the bone still leaves the periosteum to which these ligaments attach, and some bony tissue may re-grow in this area, and the process may start over again.

Osteitis Pubis

Osteitis pubis [OS-tee-i-tis Pu-bis] consists of inflammation of the *symphysis pubis*, the front middle portion of the pelvis where the pelvic wings meet. Like sacroilitis, it is usually related to pregnancy, resulting from ligamentous laxity in preparation for the pelvis to spread for delivery. It can often be very painful and lasts for quite a while, leaving some women bedridden. Oral medications of anti-inflammatory naturally are contraindicated in pregnancy, so the treatment is rest, heat, and local injections of steroids.

Chiropractic manipulation has been tried, but I have no experience with its results. X-rays, although not usually taken while pregnant, may or may not reveal changes in the pubic bones. The symptoms may last quite awhile after pregnancy, especially if bony *sclerosis* (hardening of the bone) has occurred as a result of the process.

Interestingly, an increase in the diagnosis of osteitis pubis among Australian footballers has been noticed since the sport entered the professional ranks. The amount of training and activity needed to excel in this sport—running, kicking, jumping, tackling—have all increased, placing increased stress on the pubic region. Also, the more the players exercise their abdominal musculature while training, the more stresses are directed at pubic bones. I understand that injections of local anesthetic and glucose have helped some players return to the sport.

Meralgia Paresthetica

Meralgia paresthetica [MER-al-ja PAIR-es-thet-ik-a] is as a result of impingement or compression of the *lateral cutaneous nerve* as it exits the pelvis. This nerve gives sensation over the front and outside skin of the thigh. It can present initially with a dull ache, itching, numbness, tingling, or a burning sensation over the lateral and *antero-lateral* (front and outside) thigh. The pain can be bearable but can increase in severity with time.

It affects men more than women and may involve both sides. Clinically, the history may reveal that the pain is increased by extension of the leg at the hip as well as long periods of standing or walking and is relieved by flexion of the hip.

Since this nerve is an offshoot of the L4 nerve, an L3-4 disc herniation must be ruled out, along with tumorous and infectious diseases. Conservative treatments and physical therapy, including massage and electrical stimulation, may help, but surgical intervention to decompress the nerve may be needed.

The Hip

Osteoarthritis of the Hip

The primary *etiology*, or cause, of this disease is also unknown. Internal joint injuries, dislocations, aseptic necrosis of the femoral head, and rheumatoid arthritis can lead to *osteoarthritis* (O-A) of the hip. The mechanism described for arthritis of the shoulder is probably the same here. To date, no one has found the reason for the initiation of the process.

The hip is a true ball-and-socket joint and, as discussed, is very stable. The ball at the top of the thigh bone, the *femur*, is known as the *femoral head*, and it articulates with the portion of the pelvis known as the *acetabulum* or socket. The bony portion below the femoral head is the *femoral neck*. The large winglike structure lateral to the femoral neck is known as the *greater trochanter* (Fig. 44). The major muscles from the pelvis to the hip insert here, stabilizing the pelvis with the lower leg so we don't walk with a limp. A good deal of motion is allowed with this specific construct, including flexion, extension, and internal and external rotation. The hip also has the ability to abduct and adduct. You saw these words in the shoulder discussion, but the hip doesn't have anywhere near the global motion of the shoulder since the ball is confined within the socket.

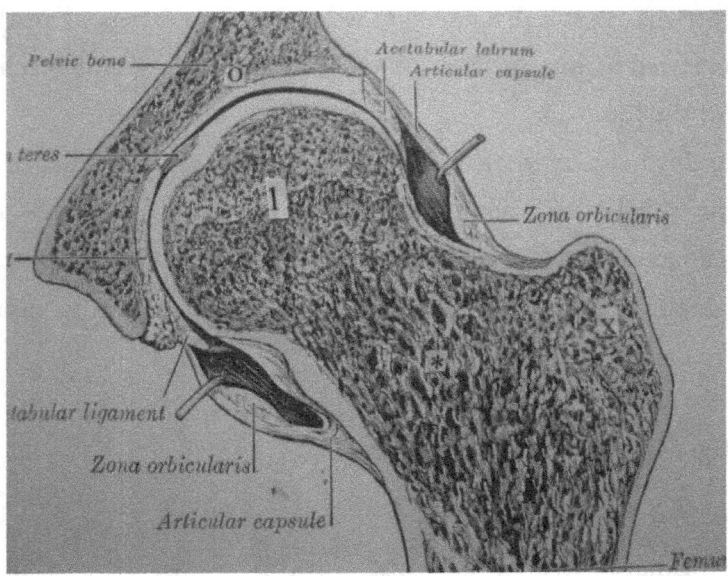

Fig. 44: Cross section of the hip joint: greater trochanter (x), femoral head (1), femoral neck. (*), Acetabulum, or hip socket (o).
Gray's Anatomy 1966

Pain from hip-joint pathology is usually present in the groin area, not in the buttock or on the outside of the thigh bone. Many patients believe any pain in their buttock is hip pain, and this is incorrect. Buttock pain is usually related to conditions of the lumbo-sacral spine. True hip pain is often referred to the groin and anterior thigh and sometimes solely to the knee joint. Many a knee has been injected, and even operated on, because of the hip's referred pain to the knee. That is why a full examination of the hip is necessary when a patient, especially a child, complains of knee pain.

Patients with hip O-A will gradually develop a limp, often throwing their body over the affected side to compensate for a weak and shortened muscular stabilizer of the hip, the *gluteus medius* [GLUE-tee-us MEE-dee-us]. They also walk with a stiff hip gait, not swinging their leg far in front of them as they walk. This is due to the loss of motion, resulting from the ball and socket's bony deformities and the tight ligaments about the joint (Fig. 45).

On examination in the *supine position*, on one's back, the thigh may no longer lie flat on the table without the pelvis rocking up. The hip cannot extend fully because of the loss of motion secondary to the tight ligaments, *flexion contracture*. It also loses its ability to rotate, and patients will have difficulty putting on socks and shoes as well as crossing their legs.

When conservative treatment fails, surgery to replace the hip joint can be a very satisfying and life-changing procedure. Most surgeons are performing total hip replacements, and recently others have begun to use a resurfacing procedure (Fig. 47), especially for the younger patient. The results of the resurfacing operations aren't all in yet, so we need to wait to see how the patients fare over time. When I performed the operation, I replaced the joint, using a plastic socket and a metal ball atop a metal prosthesis that fit into the upper thigh bone

(Fig. 46). The results are very satisfying for both the patient and the physician.

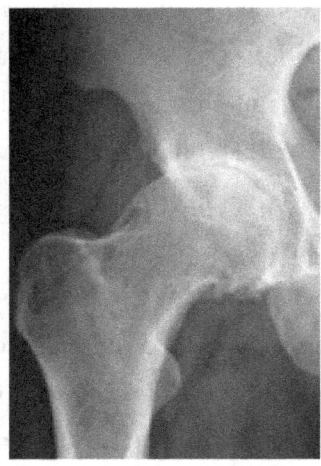

Fig. 45: Osteoarthritis of the hip: note the deformity of the ball, spurs, and cysts (dark areas in the bone) formation and loss of joint space

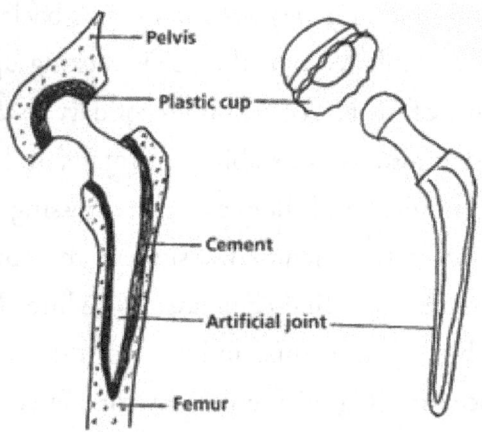

Fig. 46: One type of metal prosthesis and plastic socket, right, placed in the pelvis and femur, left. www.chesterfieldroyal.nhs.uk

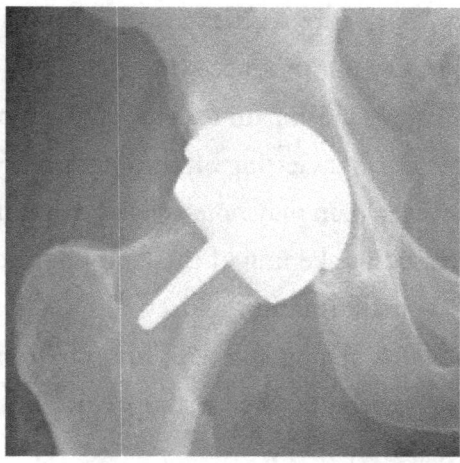

Fig. 47: Resurfaced hip joint: metal covering of ball articulates with plastic cup inside a metal socket.

Avascular Necrosis of the Hip (AVN)

This condition, known also as *osteonecrosis* [OS-te-o-nek-crow-sis] or *aseptic necrosis*, is the death of a segment of bone caused by an impaired or total loss of blood supply. It is most commonly found in the hip's femoral head, but the humeral head of the shoulder and parts of the elbow, the wrist, the knee, the ankle, and even the second metatarsal bone of the foot can be affected in one way or another. The cause is usually idiopathic, if no injury is suspected. A history of high doses of corticosteroids for various disease processes, alcoholism, AIDS, blood-clotting disorders, sickle-cell disease, liver disease, tumors, Gaucher's disease, radiation therapy, and decompression sickness may be associated with this process.

In theory, more than half the patients with avascular necrosis of one hip will develop it on the opposite side. On the injury side, a fracture of the femoral neck, even if operated on and surgically stabilized and hip dislocations can lead to AVN.

Once the process starts, a gradual deterioration inside the femoral head begins, breaking down the *medullary bone*, the soft bony structure that supports the *cortical bone* (the hard exterior bone). Tiny micro-fractures begin, which may or may not produce symptoms (Fig. 48).

The main complaint is groin pain or referred pain to the thigh or knee, especially on weight-bearing. Getting off the affected extremity will usually reduce the pain; however, pain may not occur until a collapse of the cortical bone from the increased weakening of the femoral head's bony structures. Collapse will lead to malformation and eventual arthritis or subsequent complete fracture of the femoral neck. This progression can take years or only a brief time. By the time an orthopaedist sees the patient, some collapse may be revealed by X-ray.

X-rays of the hip usually show this osteonecrosis unless the disorder is in its earliest stages. If X-rays appear to be normal, an MRI or a bone scan may be advised. If doctors discover non-traumatic osteonecrosis in one hip, they should also examine the other hip with an X-ray or an MRI.

Conservative treatment with medications for pain, crutches, avoidance of weight-bearing, and education can alleviate the pain. These measures may be adequate for treatment of the shoulder, the knee, and very small areas of avascular necrosis of the hip that may eventually heal without treatment. The body can institute its own defense against AVN, attack and absorb the dead tissue, and replace it through new vessel growth and boney support; however, with larger areas of necrosis and weight-bearing of the hip, surgical intervention is warranted.

If the cortical bone is fully intact and no fractures are evident, a *core decompression*—a hollowing out of a core of bone from the outside of the hip—from the greater trochanter into the femoral head may relieve pain and stimulate healing and offer a chance of avoiding collapse and a total hip replacement in the future. A total joint replacement or other type of joint replacement procedure seems to be the only effective procedure to relieve pain and restore motion, if osteonecrosis has caused significant bone collapse and subsequent arthritis.

A high percentage of people benefit from replacement of the hip. Total hip replacements usually last from fifteen to twenty years. When younger patients develop this disease, other techniques are usually attempted to avoid total replacement because replacements may have to be revised or totally replaced at some later time.

Some physicians perform a newer technique of surface replacement arthroplasty to treat osteonecrosis of the hip in younger people. This procedure involves placing a metal cap over the femoral head rather than replacing the entire joint, as is done in a standard total hip replacement. If the hip socket also is involved, a second metal cap is placed in the socket. It is not clear whether surface replacement arthroplasty is better than standard hip replacement, and results of these operations are currently being evaluated.

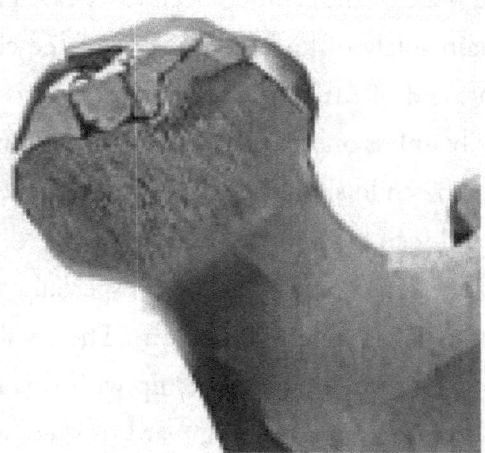

Fig. 48: Diagram of avascular necrosis of the femoral head with micro-fractures
Image courtesy of Medical Multimedia Group LLC, www.eorthopod.com

Slipped Capital Femoral Epiphysis

All bones grow from cartilaginous forms. Once the major portion of this formation *ossifies* or becomes bone, growth occurs at the end of long bones from an area called an *epiphysis* [eh-PIF-fis-sis]. In the growing child, it is separated from the rest of the bone by a special cartilage junction that allows for growth. In adults, this growth center disappears and is replaced by bone.

There are two relatively common conditions found in the femoral head: *slipped capital femoral epiphysis* (SCFE) and *Legg-Calvé-Perthes disease*. These occur in children and must be recognized as quickly as possible before deformity occurs.

With a SCFE, the growth center of the femur at the hip joint can loosen and actually allow the top of the femoral head to slip off the femur neck like melting ice cream slipping off a cone. Initially, a *pre-slip* can occur where X-rays are normal, but the child complains of groin and thigh pain. Occasionally, one may see a slight widening of the cartilage between the epiphysis and the bone of the femoral neck by X-ray. They can, as already discussed, complain solely of knee pain. Most of the children I saw were males, overweight, and of Afro-American descent. This pre-slip condition can be missed easily unless one is well aware of its existence in children and its repercussions. The child should be placed on crutches and refrain from bearing weight until seen by an orthopaedist.

On examination, some pain is elicited, especially when rotating the thigh inward on the pelvis (internal rotation). There will also be some loss of motion and possibly spasm about the hip with this maneuver. The leg involved may be shorter and rotated outward. If there is any concern that this may be the diagnosis, immediate surgery to pin—the slipped portion in place—is necessary since continued slippage of the epiphysis off the femur will deform the ball and cause arthritis in the future. Some orthopaedists believe the other hip should be operated on soon thereafter since there is an increased risk of the opposite hip being affected statistically.

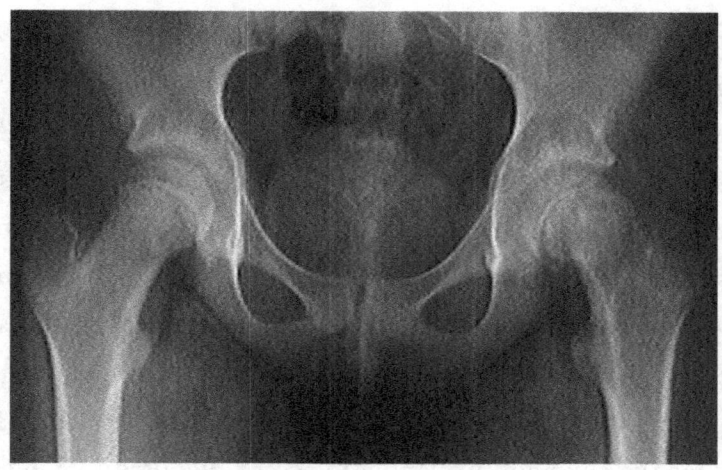

Fig. 49: Slipped capital femoral epiphysis on the right: Note how the round top of the femoral head has slipped down and counterclockwise compared with the quarter moon top of the femoral head on the left.

When the epiphysis does slip off, varying degrees of slippage can be present. When I was dealing with these conditions, any slip was pinned *in situ* (as it was found), and any resultant deformity was dealt with at a later time, if necessary. Once the slip had healed, cutting the upper femur bone—an *osteotomy*—to reposition the ball as correctly anatomical as possible to its original articulation with the socket could be performed. I believe this policy still holds today.

One may ask what effect this surgery has on the epiphysis' ability to add to the growth of the entire femur itself. Luckily, 80 percent of the growth of the femur comes from the knee end, so the length of the femur is not overly affected by the slip and the subsequent closure of the growth center from the surgery.

It is very important to remember that any child from ages ten to fifteen complaining of groin, thigh, or knee pain without injury should be examined for a slipped capital femoral epiphysis, especially if the patient is male, black, and overweight.

Legg-Calvé-Perthes Disease

Legg-Calvé-Perthes disease is not a common disease of the hip. It occurs predominately in males between two and twelve years old, most patients being in the first decade of life. There is no etiology of this disease; however, some form of blood supply interruption to the proximal bony epiphysis of the femur occurs, causing death of the bone (*osteonecrosis*) leading to micro-fractures of the bone. The body then attempts to heal this process by absorbing the bony fragmentation and rebuilding it. This process takes years to occur and can be very difficult to treat as well as difficult for the child and his family to accept. We used to apply casts to the child's legs with a wooden strut between the legs to hold the thighs out. This would place the entire femoral head inside the socket to help prevent malformation and compression from the edges of the socket. You would think this treatment would slow children down, but many of these kids could fly down corridors in our clinic with the use of their crutches. It was an amazing sight to behold.

If the body cannot adequately rebuild the epiphysis, deformity and arthritis may occur later. Ultimately, arthritis may necessitate hip replacement in adulthood.

Transient Synovitis of the Hip

Transient synovitis of the hip joint is a condition that causes hip pain during childhood. The cause of transient synovitis is not known, but it may be related to a viral illness. Transient synovitis tends to occur from ages two to nine and causes inflammation and pain around the hip joint. Usually, the child will refuse to bear weight on the lower extremity, often crying when doing so. The symptoms tend to begin quickly and resolve soon thereafter, often after a viral illness. Findings include pain with movement of the hip joint, hip and knee pain complaints, difficulty with walking on the extremity, and low-grade fever.

This diagnosis has findings very similar to those of a septic or infected hip joint, so it is imperative to watch for the worsening symptoms of a possible bacterial infection. If the two diagnoses cannot be differentiated, an aspiration of the hip may be necessary to make the proper diagnosis. The infected hip will identify pus in the *aspirate* (fluid removed), whereas the hip involved with transient synovitis will not.

In many children with possible transient synovitis, a period of observation in the hospital or emergency room is sufficient to make the diagnosis. Children who have a septic (infected) hip tend to rapidly worsen. Children with transient synovitis improve over time. If the diagnosis is transient synovitis, the most important aspect of treatment is time. Parents should keep tabs on any fever, especially if the temperature steadily increases.

Transient synovitis of the hip usually results in complete recovery. An infected hip joint can be a medical emergency, so any worsening hip symptoms involving fever must be evaluated immediately.

Greater Trochanteric Bursitis

The *greater trochanteric bursa* is located under a large, flat tendon on the outside or lateral portion of the hip area (Fig. 50) and the outside edge of the greater trochanter. It is probably the largest bursa in the body. Its primary function, as with all bursae, is to reduce friction as the flat tendon—the *ilio-tibial band of the fascia* [FAS-sha] *lata*—courses over the greater trochanter. This large bony winglike structure is located at the top of the femur bone lateral to the femoral head and neck. The gluteus medius and minimus muscles attach here, balancing the pelvis so we can walk without limping or throwing our center of gravity over our hip.

Inflammation of this bursa occurs often but can be difficult to diagnose unless the physician listens carefully to the patient and asks the most important question of all: "Where is the pain? Point to exactly where you feel the pain." Whether or not the pain is referred makes no difference as long as the patient points to one area because the pain is either there or referred, and if one knows the referral patterns, the diagnosis can be made. Pressing on the area and eliciting the pain the patient describes usually means the pain is in that specific area. This is not always true, if you remember the tender area of the trapezius muscle with degenerative neck disc's referred pain.

In my experience, the usual conservative measures don't do much for this condition, but an injection of refined steroid and a local anesthetic usually relieves the symptoms. Several injections may be needed. I used to lay the patient on his side, placing a large pillow between his legs with the hip slightly flexed to relax the tension on the ilio-tibial band. Having identified the most tender area and swabbed the area with antiseptic solution, I would introduce the needle through the skin and the ilio-tibial band until I was under it. The physician can feel the needle penetrate this thick tendon. I would then inject the fluid in four directions, trying to dissipate the fluid throughout the entire bursa. One should never feel resistance to the flow of this injection. If one does, the needle is not in the correct spot.

Should the injection not eliminate all the pain within a few minutes, the inflammation may have scarred the bursa, not allowing the free flow of the fluid. That is why another one or two injections in different areas may be needed at the next visit.

Incidentally, when this bursitis is a result of an injury, it is usually because the patient has fallen directly upon the greater trochanter area, acutely compressing the bursa. The bursa responds to the injury with acute inflammation and swelling. Athletes name this injury a *hip pointer*.

Snapping Hip Syndrome

This is a hodgepodge of conditions that create a snapping sound or feeling about the hip. The problem may be inside the joint (*intra-articular*) or outside (*extra-articular*). The intra-articular lesions are less common than those outside the joint. The hip joint may have a loose body or torn cartilage (*labrum*), similar to that of the shoulder that moves to and fro. The conditions outside are either medial or lateral. On the lateral side, the most common is the fascia lata tendon flipping over the greater trochanter, and on the medial side, it's the ilio-psoas tendon sliding back and forth on the inside of the femoral neck as the patient's flexes and extends his hip. Pain is usually not a sign unless the bursae in these areas become inflamed enough. These snapping episodes may disappear after awhile, but if no pain is associated with them, only conservative treatment is advised. Surgery is usually not suggested unless there is an intra-articular problem that may cause a permanent or progressive arthritic condition in the future.

Ilio-Psoas Bursitis

This can be a tricky diagnosis to make. I believe an iliopsoas [*Ill*-e-o-sow-as] bursitis is more prevalent in one's orthopaedic practice than realized. Its pain is almost identical to the pain of hip arthritis, but the motion of the hip is not usually affected on physical exam. The ilio-psoas muscle originates in the pelvis and inserts on the *lesser trochanter of the upper femur*, a small bony protrusion on the inner posterior aspect of the femur just below the hip joint. This muscle flexes the hip and slightly rotates the femur outward. There is a small bursa in this area between the tendon and the bone that allows the tendon to glide smoothly as it flexes the hip (Fig. 50). Inflammation of this bursa can occur, especially with over-exercising of the hip. Many cases occur for no reason at all.

I usually diagnosed this condition by first noting that the hip-joint motion is not affected while passively placing the hip through its range of motion. With the patient supine, hip flexed, and fully rotated outward (*externally rotated*), I pressed directly on the area of the bursa and asked the patient to lift his leg upward and inward. This maneuver should reproduce the pain of the bursitis.

Again, conservative measures may fail, and an injection may be necessary. An injection here is not as easy as in other areas since important structures are present nearby such as the femoral artery, vein, and the femoral nerve. These structures are usually lateral—to the right of the right ilio-psoas bursa and to the left of the left bursa—when injecting with the hip slightly flexed and fully rotated outward. Needless to say, this injection should be done carefully and under the supervision of a physician knowledgeable in the hip's anatomy.

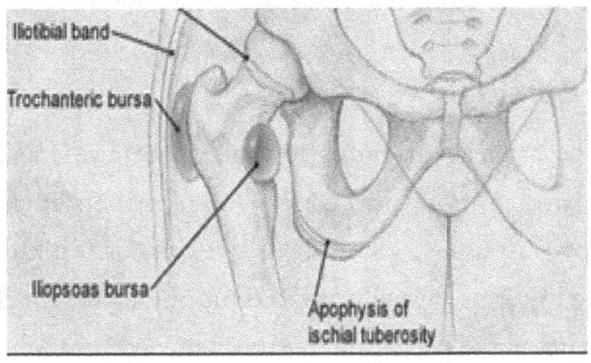

Fig. 50: Greater trochanteric bursa, the ilio-psoas bursa, and ischial tuberosity. Inferior pubic ramus (x)
www.handbook.muh.ie

Ischial Tuberosity Bursitis

The *ischial tuberosity* [Ish-e-al tube-er-OSS-it-tee] is the lower portion of the pelvis, on which we sit. (Fig. 50). The bursa protecting this area occasionally becomes inflamed and causes another real "pain in the rear." I mention this bursitis, not because it is a common condition, but because its pain can be confused with that of herniated lumbar discs and the pain of spinal stenosis. Exquisite tenderness and reproduction of the patient's pain over the ischial spine confirms the diagnosis. The common bursitis treatments above are used for this process as well.

Groin Pulls and Hamstring Tears

These are common injuries among athletes. Several muscles, large and small, are attached from the pelvis to the femur bone. These areas of the pelvis are called the *pubis bone* and its *inferior ramus*, the front right or left portion of the pelvis and their extensions downward (Fig. 50). These muscles can be strained, partially torn, or completely torn, causing pain in the groin area (*groin pulls*), along with inability to flex or extend the hip well.

The hamstring muscles are the muscles in the back of the thigh. They originate from the ischial tuberosity of the pelvis (Fig. 50) and extend down the back of the thigh to the back of the knee. These muscles help extend the hip, especially when running. You will often see an athlete pull up after running a distance and hold the back of his thigh. One or more of the hamstring muscles have been strained, partially torn, or ruptured.

When a muscle is strained, its fibers mostly remain intact, so its recovery is relatively short. When the muscle partially tears, some of its fibers tear apart, and some fibers remain intact. The healing process here is longer. When the muscle fully tears or ruptures from the pelvis or in the main body of the muscle, the healing process can be very long, sometimes ending some athletes' careers.

Muscles that rupture heal only by way of scar tissue formed by the blood from the initial injury. The area of rupture does not reproduce more muscle fibers. The blood clots form fibrous tissue and eventually scar that contracts. Rehabilitation for such injuries eventually treats the tight scar with stretching exercises; however, there always exists a muscle-scar tissue interval on both sides of the initial rupture that is subject to re-injury. That is why professional football players can be plagued by groin and hamstring tears for many years and often end their careers because of them. It is imperative that the first injury of this sort be treated very conservatively, leaving much time for the healing process to occur. Returning to the field of play too soon may be a very big mistake.

Thigh and Hip Contusions and Hematomas

A *contusion* is bleeding into the skin as a result of a compressive injury or external blow. These injuries almost always follow a fall or a blow from without, especially about the buttock, the outer hip area, or thigh. Actually, they can occur anywhere. The force of the fall compresses the skin tissue, rupturing small blood vessels in the superficial tissue below the skin. Depending on the force and the area involved, the contusion could be mild or severe. The skin will turn black and blue, known as *ecchymosis* [ECK-key-mo-sis]. More severe forces may involve the small vessels deep within the subcutaneous or *adipose* (fatty) tissue just below the skin. Blood in this area can eventually reach skin level and presents as a black and blue mark as well. A large bleed within the fatty tissue can present as a ballooning of this area, with much pain and ecchymosis consistent with a *hematoma* [HE-ma-toe-ma], a collection of blood caused by much bleeding into any tissue or space. Some hematomas can be enormous and quite impressive on presentation.

Initially, ice, rest, and time are the main treatments for these entities. Most hematomas will be absorbed by the body over time, but some will not. The blood clot that is produced may well be too large for the body to handle. *Aspiration*, pulling the blood out with a needle and syringe, may decrease the size of the blood collection enough to allow the body to absorb the rest. For very large hematomas, a surgical evacuation of the blood clot may be necessary.

Resolving hematomas should be carefully watched. Occasionally, bacteria find their way to this area, and since there is little, if any, oxygen present in a blood clot, the bacteria can multiply and develop into a serious infection.

Falls and external blows from sports may create hematoma formation within muscles. This is a more serious injury. A mild to moderate bleed within the muscle may stop purely by its own pressure buildup within the muscle, a *tamponade effect*; however, some bleeds continue, causing abnormal pressures within the muscle, enough to cause the muscle to die. Immediate surgery is necessary to decompress the muscle before this can occur. This procedure is known as a *fasciotomy* [FAS-she-ot-o-me] and involves surgically incising the lining about the muscle to relieve the muscle of the blood clot pressure. This often occurs in the calf, where there are multiple compartments of muscles. This will be discussed at length in chapter 16.

CHAPTER 14
THE KNEE

The knee is more complicated than most folks realize. Sure, it bends and straightens or, as we orthopaedists say, flexes and extends. That's a given, but did you know that, to some degree, a normal knee rotates? Let's take a look at its anatomy.

Two long bones of the leg meet to form the knee: the lower end of the thigh bone, or femur (Fig. 51A), and the flattened top of one of the lower leg bones, the *tibia* [TIB-ee-ya] (Fig. 51A). At the point where these bones meet, each is shaped to fit into and glide over the other bone like parts of a 3-D puzzle. The end of the femur has two large knoblike protrusions (the *femoral condyles* [KON-dials]), while the top of the tibia (the *tibial plateau*) has two indentations that correspond to and fit the femoral condyles perfectly, so the tibia rotates and glides on femur when it flexes or extends.

These corresponding parts are formed in a way that allows the tibia to actually rotate and lock on the condyles when the knee is virtually straight. This *screw-home mechanism* enables us to stand on one leg with the knee fully extended without using our muscles to hold that position. Before vaccines put an end to poliomyelitis, folks whose legs had been paralyzed by the disease could still stand and walk by locking their knees in this manner.

Ligaments hold the femur and tibia together, the major ones being the *medial collateral ligament*, the *lateral collateral ligament*, and the *anterior and posterior cruciate* [KRU-she-et] *ligaments* (Fig. 51A). The medial collateral ligament connects the inside of the femur to the tibia. The lateral collateral ligament connects the outside femur to the fibula. The fibula is also connected to the outside portion of the tibia by short, hefty ligaments. The anterior and posterior cruciate ligaments, which lie between the two indentations of the tibial plateau and in the notch between the femoral condyles (Fig. 51A), effectively prevent forward or backward displacement of the tibia on the femur.

A

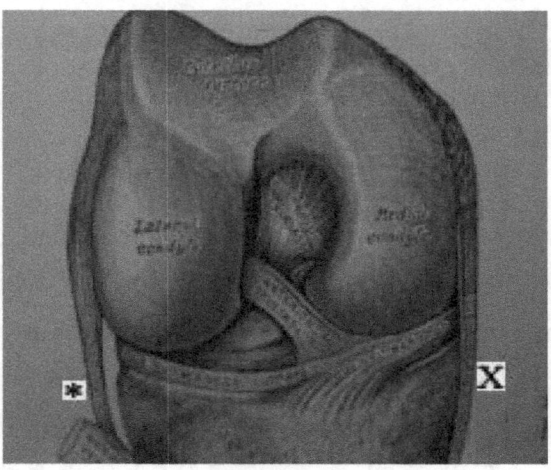

Fig. 51A: The right knee viewed from the front: note the femoral condyles, upside-down U shape inter-condylar notch, anterior and posterior cruciate ligaments crossing each other in the inter-condylar notch, medial collateral ligament (x) and lateral collateral ligament (*).

B

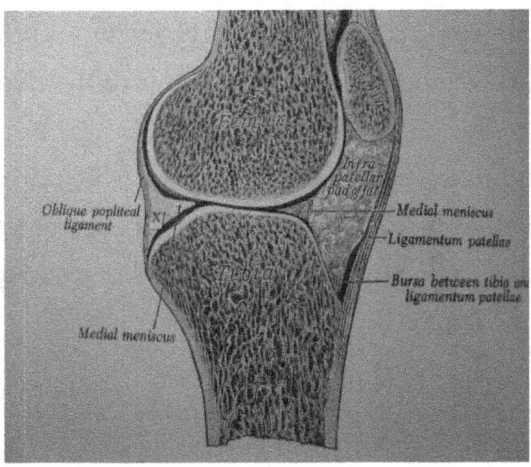

Fig. 51B: Cross section of knee joint from the side. Note the pie-shaped meniscus on the left (x) and front of the knee; the quadriceps tendon above the kneecap (patella), patellar tendon below the patella, and the patellar fat pad, behind the patellar tendon.
Gray's Anatomy, 1966

The major muscle mass on the front of the thigh, the *quadriceps*, straightens the knee. The quadriceps (Latin for *four heads*) is so named because it comprises four muscles. The quadriceps muscles transition to a thick short tendon (the *quadriceps tendon*) as they insert into the top of the kneecap (the *patella*), which glides on the femur beneath it (Fig. 51B). A tendon arising from the bottom portion of the kneecap (the *patellar tendon*) eventually attaches to the upper front aspect of the tibia. When the quadriceps contracts, it pulls the tibia up to straighten or extend the knee. Other muscles on the back of the thigh are active in flexing the knee. These are known as *hamstring* muscles.

Inside the knee, each femoral condyle is cushioned by a fibrous disc of fibrocartilage, a *meniscus* [Men-is-cus]—the medial meniscus on the inner side, and the lateral meniscus on the outer. When the femoral condyles press against the tibial plateau, these two fibrous discs provide resilience and support. Altogether, they can carry up to 85 percent of the load on the knee, so keeping these discs intact is very important to the knee's function.

Like all joint surfaces, the condyles and the tibial plateau have a covering of hyaline cartilage, the smooth, glistening white material I've discussed that reduces friction as bones glide over each other. The synovial fluid nourishes each meniscus in the absence of a true blood supply as well as the hyaline cartilage covering of the bones.

Most folks have heard the term "*torn cartilage in the knee*." This term is usually applied to a torn meniscus, either medial or lateral, rather than the hyaline cartilage on the ends of bones that constitute a joint surface. For the rest of this chapter, rather than calling it a *cartilage*, I will use the term *meniscus* or its plural, *menisci*. The diagram in Fig. 52 shows a bird's eyeview of the positions of the menisci on the tibial plateau.

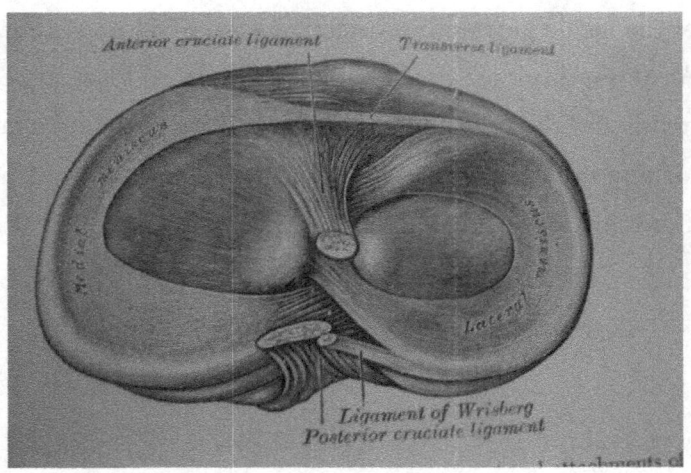

Fig. 52: Left knee: looking down on top of the tibial plateau.
Lateral meniscus on the right and medial meniscus on the left:
the two cross sectioned ligaments in the center are the anterior cruciate ligament and the posterior cruciate ligament.
Gray's Anatomy, 1966

Knee Injuries

Meniscus Tears

A meniscus can be torn in various ways: twisting, hyperflexion (extreme bending) of the knee, or hyperextension (straightening beyond the normal range) of the knee. The most common cause is a twisting injury, the medial meniscus usually being the one torn. This can happen with no damage whatsoever to any ligaments. Several types of tears can occur.

- The meniscus may be torn from its moorings around the edges or near the edges longitudinally (Fig. 53)
- It can be split obliquely so there is a loose piece at one end, with the other end still attached, known as a *flap tear* (Fig. 54)
- The middle of the meniscus can split, a *longitudinal tear*
- A longitudinal tear long enough to permit looseness and mobility of the inside portion can occur, a *bucket-handle tear* (Fig. 54).
- At times, this loose portion may be displaced forward between the femur and the tibia and be caught in front of the femoral condyle, locking the knee so it can't fully extend (Fig. 55)
- Combinations of these can occur.

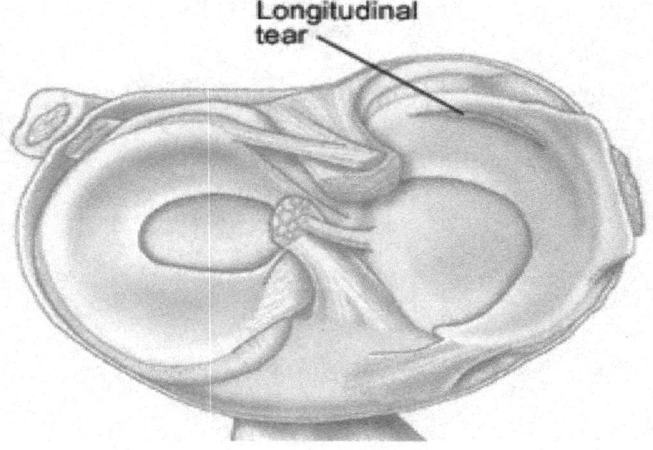

Fig. 53: Peripheral meniscus tear
www.yorkshirekneeclinic.com

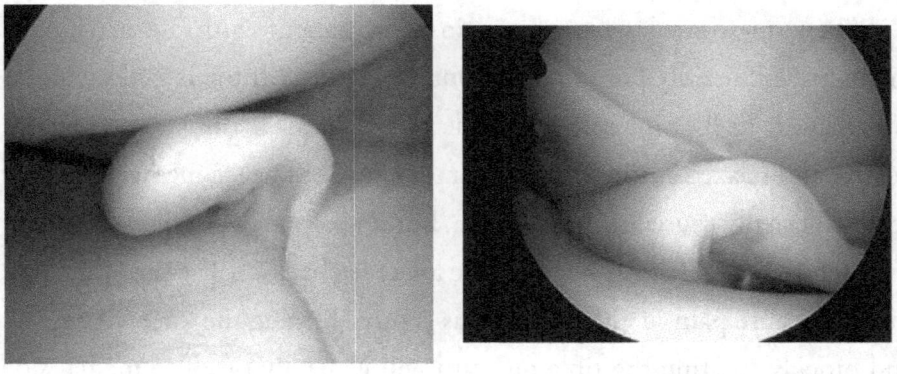

Fig. 54: Flap tear of a meniscus visualized at arthroscopy
www.yorkshirekneeclinic.com

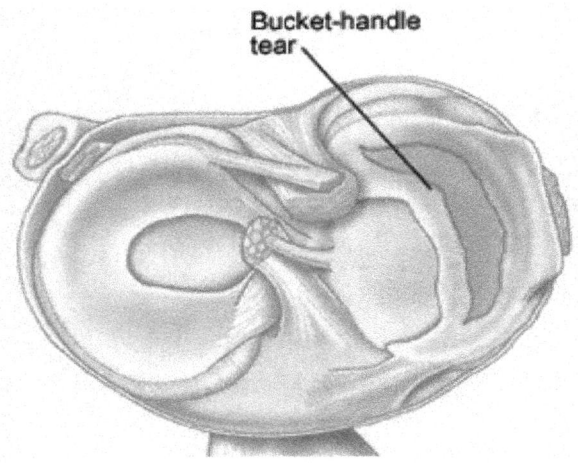

Fig. 55: Arthroscopic photo of loose piece of tear, dislocated in front of condyle, locking knee in flexed position.
Below it : Diagram of bucket-handle tear of meniscus.
www.yorkshirekneeclinic.com

When questioned where his pain is, a patient with a torn medial meniscus will usually point to the front inside knee. If the lateral meniscus is damaged, he'll point to the outside of the knee. If the person remains passive and relaxed as the physician straightens the knee, a medial meniscus tear will usually cause immediate pain, but no pain may be felt if the lateral meniscus is torn. Quickly bending the lower leg backward against the thigh may also cause pain, if either meniscus is torn. Flexing the knee 90 degrees and quickly rotating the tibia outward will generally produce medial side pain of a medial meniscus tear, and twisting quickly inward may produce typical lateral meniscus pain. Also, if the medial meniscus is torn, the medial joint line will be tender as the doctor presses from front to back. The same is true if the lateral joint line is examined by pressing for lateral meniscus tenderness. The *joint line* is that area on the side of the knee where the femur and the tibia meet. The medial joint line is on the inside, and the lateral joint line is on the outside of the knee.

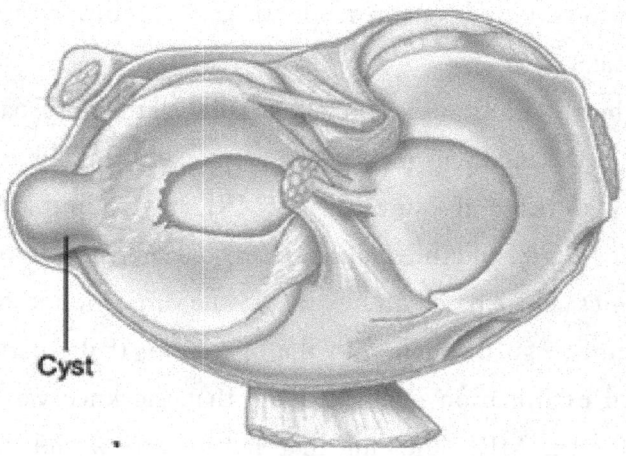

Fig. 56: Lateral meniscus cyst. Note degenerative changes of the meniscus in this area as well.
www.yorkshirekneeclinic.com

A lateral joint line that feels larger or thicker than normal and even bulging represents a collection of fluid, or a *lateral meniscal cyst*, a sure indicator of a lateral meniscus degeneration or tear (Fig. 56). Horizontal splitting of the lateral meniscus as it tears allows fluid from the joint to flow through the split and accumulate outside the joint. This finding is rare with tears of the medial meniscus. Fluid may also be present in the knee after any meniscus tear. With the leg lying straight on the examining table, the physician will sometimes cup the sides of the joint with both hands and compress the knee to try to force any fluid upward in the knee. He will then try to bounce the kneecap up and down. If fluid is present, the kneecap will be easily pressed down and then pop up.

When the edges of a meniscus pull away from its attachments to ligaments, chances of its healing on its own are good as it still has a true blood supply. If a meniscus tear is more central, however, the lack of any blood supply will prevent healing. Such a tear will remain partially detached for a long time, causing the knee to lock, snap, or give way. If it interferes with the person's lifestyle, arthroscopic surgery is indicated to remove the loose material.

Although an MRI examination will usually tell the physician where and how much of the meniscus is torn, the study is not infallible. I have seen what seemed to be an absolute tear on MRI only to find an undamaged knee joint at surgery, and the opposite has also been true. Ultimately, it will be the patient's choice based on his trust in the surgeon, not the MRI, that persuades him to go through with the operation. If the patient's history and physical examination convinced me that the knee was damaged, I often skipped the MRI, knowing that arthroscopy would tell me much more about the structures inside the knee.

Arthroscopic surgery begins with small incisions, or *portals*, made in the knee, usually one on either side of the kneecap tendon. After filling the joint with fluid, the surgeon introduces a combined scope and camera that's connected to a television monitor. He then carries out a thorough examination. A second portal allows him to introduce instruments to probe the soft tissues, find the problem, and decide on a method for removing loose material, whether by using shavers, cutters, lasers, or coagulators. Removal of the meniscus is known as a *meniscectomy* [men-is-SECK-tuh-me]. The operation ends with the suturing of the skin over the portals and the bandaging of the knee. Rehabilitation after a meniscectomy is quite short as only loose material is removed, with no reconstruction necessary.

If during the procedure, on the other hand, the surgeon finds that the tear has a good enough blood supply to heal, rather than simply removing the meniscus, he may repair the tear. He does this by trimming the two pieces of the tear so that they will fit well together, shaves the outside portion to a bleeding base, and connects the two pieces using either sutures or bio-absorbable material (Fig. 57). Some postoperative immobilization is necessary as the repaired fragments heal together. Chances of healing will be high, if a good blood supply is restored to the damaged meniscus.

Even in cases where blood supply is questionable, most surgeons proceed with the repair, especially in younger patients, hoping the meniscus will heal. Success in these cases may be less likely, and another operation to remove the offending piece may be necessary.

Why do we attempt the repair in such cases? The meniscus is extremely important as a cushion for the condyles and support for the knee. Removing all or even just some of it may predispose the bone ends to eventual arthritic changes. Therefore, if the surgeon believes healing of the tear is possible, he will carry out the repair.

Patient and doctor should discuss all these factors at length before any decision is made about surgery, giving much weight to the patient's feelings and desires. For some folks, a disrupted lifestyle will rule out acceptance of a repair as they want to get back on their feet soon and return to daily activities rather than be laid up during a slow rehabilitation.

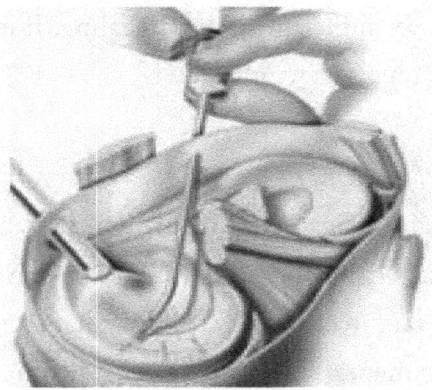

Fig. 57: Diagram of meniscus repair using bio-absorbable darts.
Note arthroscope on left.
The Knee & Shoulder Centers of NJ and PA

Ligament Injuries

Medial Collateral Ligament

The medial collateral ligament (MCL) is the main stabilizer of the knee's inner side. A direct blow from the outside is the most common cause of injury to the MCL although it can also be injured in other ways—for example, if the foot slips outward just as one begins to pivot in the opposite direction. This movement, suddenly forcing the knee into a knock-kneed position, places great stress on the inside of the knee and the MCL, causing it to stretch (grade 1), partially tear (grade 2), or fully tear (grade 3). Most MCL injuries are grade 1 or grade 2. A grade 3 injury is rare, and in this injury, other structures should tear as well.

Conservative treatment is appropriate for grades 1 and 2 injuries, which usually heal given enough time. However, because the medial meniscus is attached to the inner surface of the MCL and may have torn as well, an MRI examination may be needed to reveal the condition of the meniscus, if symptoms persist after sufficient time for healing. If it is damaged, surgery may be required to repair or remove it.

Lateral Collateral Ligament

The lateral collateral ligament (LCL), which stabilizes the outside of the knee, is much less likely than the MCL to stretch or rupture. It can be injured, however, by a force contrary to those that damage the MCL. If the posterior lateral ligaments are also involved, treating the knee's resultant instability will be difficult. With such an injury, the anterior cruciate or posterior cruciate ligament may also be damaged, a rare and difficult condition to diagnose in the acute stage. A hyperextension twisting force is thought to be the mechanism of this injury.

Anterior Cruciate Ligament Injuries

My feelings about injury to the anterior cruciate ligament (ACL) arise from both personal and professional experience because I was injured in 1955 when a defensive lineman fell on the outside of my knee, twisting it into a knock-kneed position. The injury totally ruptured my MCL (grade 3), took out my ACL, and tore my medial meniscus—the "terrible triad," as it was known in those days. I had no treatment other than rest, and in fact, I never saw an orthopaedist.

The swelling and pain eventually disappeared, but for years, I experienced multiple episodes of my knee giving way, locking, or just "not being there" for me. Orthopaedists understood little about the knee and its injuries at that time. Repairs were fraught with discouraging results. Not until I finished my orthopaedic residency and my stint in the US Navy did I begin to understand the knee's complexities. Even then, open surgery to reconstruct knees with ACL damage was still technically difficult, necessitated lengthy rehabilitation, and often resulted in a stiff and painful knee. Techniques to stabilize the ACL without replacing it evolved although they were not terribly successful and led to other problems down the road. Because my knee has undergone many degenerative changes, at some point, I will probably have a total knee replacement. What a shame that the knowledge and surgical techniques of today weren't available in 1955!

Now let's get back to the ACL. This ligament, like the posterior cruciate ligament (PCL), gets the *cruciate* in its name from the fact that the two ligaments cross within the central part of the knee. The ACL is comprised of two major bundles and a smaller third bundle. The anterior medial bundle tightens to stabilize the knee in flexion and loosens in extension; the posterior lateral bundle tightens to stabilize the knee in extension and loosens in flexion.

The ACL is injured far more often than the PCL. Both ligaments help the knee by keeping the end of the tibia from slipping on the end of the femur: the ACL prevents forward slippage; the PCL, backward slippage. Outside forces may not be the cause of an ACL injury. Many ACL ruptures occur without contact. A football player will sometimes fall to the ground suddenly for no known reason and later be found to have an ACL tear. The injury probably occurs most often as a result of running and trying to change position by planting a foot before pivoting or while decelerating. When that happens, the forward motion causes the tibia to slip on the femur, stressing and then tearing the ACL.

Soon after an acute injury, blood may collect in the knee, usually with pain, but I've seen some cases of a partly torn ACL with only discomfort and no severe pain. After the acute injury, many folks complain of a knee giving way at the same time as they feel a bone going out of place and then popping back in, especially on the outside of the knee. I know this feeling very well.

Specific physical findings are present with an ACL tear that leave no question about the diagnosis. In one test, with the knee straight, the examiner can move the upper end of the tibia upward while keeping the femur immobile (the *Lachman Test*). In another test, carried out with the knee at 90 degrees and the patient's foot on the table, the examiner can pull the upper end of the tibia forward while the femur stays in place (the *Drawer Test*). This, too, is diagnostic of an ACL tear. Finally, with the knee partly bent and the examiner holding the tibia rotated inward, a slight force is applied to establish a knock-kneed position when the knee is fully straightened. If the tibia can be felt popping into place (the *Pivot Shift Test*), there is no question that the ACL has been torn.

If these tests are all positive for an ACL tear, the doctor will usually order an MRI examination to evaluate the entire joint for any other problem. At that point, if the patient's symptoms disrupt his or her lifestyle, the decision to proceed with an ACL reconstruction is the right one. Any young athlete should have the operation to get back to full activity and avoid future knee damage. Unless an isolated ACL tear is mended, the patient is likely to experience repeated episodes of instability and risk a meniscus tear, leading to eventual arthritic changes in the joint. If there are injuries in addition to the ACL tear, they can be corrected at the same time.

Fortunately, arthroscopic-assisted surgery makes ACL reconstructions routine and quite successful overall. The surgeon will replace the ligament, either with tendon taken from the patient's own body (an *autograft*) or with freeze-dried tendon taken from a cadaver (an *allograft*). The grafts are placed in bony tunnels starting in the tibia, slid up into the knee joint, and into a tunnel in the femur (Fig. 58). Some grafts may have bone at each end. Multiple devices hold the bone and tendon in place in the tunnels or canals. Just before stabilizing the last device, the surgeon will tighten the graft to try to replicate the tension present in the original ACL, although doing so exactly may not be possible because the original ACL is comprised of two ligamentous bundles that worked in opposition. We have yet to produce a graft that can work as well as the one our Maker devised even though the so-called *double bundle technique* was developed to do so.

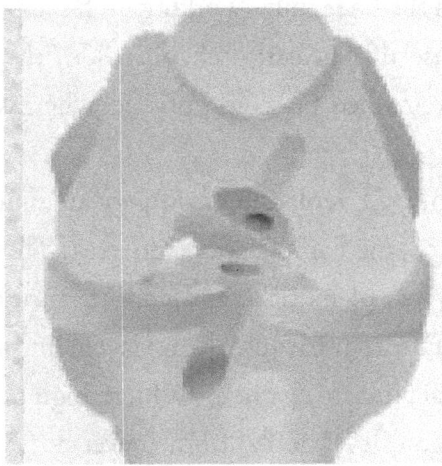

Fig. 58: Tunnels drilled in femur and tibia for the ACL grafting material
www.drmendbone.com

I first performed ACL reconstruction in the late 1980s with good to excellent results in 85–90 percent of the cases. I routinely used cadaver grafts, while most surgeons now use the patient's own tissue, either kneecap or hamstring tendons. Rebuilding the original ruptured ACL is impossible as once this short ligament tears into multiple strands like spaghetti, trying to suture them would be like trying to nail a custard pie to a wall. Surgeons attempt to position the graft in the same points of attachment to the tibia and the femur as the original ACL. This is the most technically difficult part of the procedure. A poorly aligned graft will not work well and may, in fact, ultimately fail. Therefore, much time and effort is needed to be sure the graft placement is as close to the original as possible.

The procedure I've just described requires very little immobilization of the knee afterward, and because most of the knee's motion is to be regained in the first six to eight weeks, getting the patient moving immediately is vital. I always stressed the importance of regaining full extension of the knee in early therapy because postoperative bleeding in the operative site will form clots and then a dense scar tissue that physically blocks one's ability to straighten the knee fully. Working on full extension was foremost in my mind because during early rehabilitation, this clot and resultant fibrous scar tissue remained loose and pliable, whereas later, they become more rigid.

Complications of ACL replacement surgery are much fewer today than they once were, but some complications do exist. They include infection, residual instability, loss of motion, and another rupture. Re-ruptures are not common but may occur because the replacement tissues are often not a strong as the original cruciate ligament. While a high percentage of patients return to their previous level of play, some never do.

Knee Dislocations

A *total dislocation of the knee* is a true orthopaedic emergency. If the femur separates totally from the tibia, some—if not all—of the major ligaments of the knee will have ruptured, and nerves as well as an important artery in the back of the knee may have been damaged.

The dislocation must be addressed immediately by manipulating the bones back into place and conducting specific studies to evaluate the status of the *popliteal* [pop-lie-TEE-al] *artery*, the blood vessel in the back of the knee that supplies blood to the lower leg and foot. These studies should include an *arteriogram* [ar-TEER-ee-oh-gram], an X-ray study with injection of fluid (*contrast material*) that will be visible on X-ray, into the femoral artery in the groin to be observed as it flows down the leg. If any of the fluid appears not to be flowing through the artery, or if it spreads outside it, a vascular surgeon will be called in immediately for the crucial repair of this important blood vessel. Because the nerves to the lower leg and foot may also be stretched or torn, continued monitoring of these structures is essential, with surgery to repair them, if necessary.

Recovery from such an injury may take years. Fortunately, an orthopaedist will see very few such injuries in the course of a career. I was on call one night when a young girl was brought in with total dislocations of both knees. A car had hit her while she tried to rescue an opossum in the road. (As it turned out, the opossum was already dead, so her efforts were in vain.) After a vascular surgeon repaired both popliteal arteries, my partner and I worked for eight hours to complete the reconstruction. She had a satisfactory early result in that she could walk, but I never knew the final outcome as she never returned to my office once the acute care phase had passed.

Other Knee Conditions

Loose Bodies

So-called *loose bodies* of the knee can appear without the presence of any other disorder. Where they come from is often a puzzle, and they can be very easy or very difficult to diagnose. Someone may complain of a movable lump inside the knee and, when asked to demonstrate it, moves the leg into a certain position and feels around until the loose body slides under his finger. If the doctor puts his hand in the same place, he may also feel the loose body. This typically happens if the loose body works its way into the *suprapatellar* [sou-prah-pa-TELL-ar] *pouch*, the area of the joint above and behind the kneecap. Sometimes, an X-ray may show a loose body but only if it has calcified.

An easy diagnosis? Well, no. Many loose bodies don't behave in this way. The patient may feel the lump once in a while, but he can't do it predictably and particularly not in the doctor's office. He may complain only of something catching in his knee and a feeling of the knee giving way. A snapping sound may be the only symptom. X-rays may not reveal anything because the loose body isn't calcified and consists only of cartilage that doesn't show up on X-ray.

The patient wants answers, so what's the physician going to do, order an MRI? Possibly, but it may not reveal anything. A computer-assisted tomography (CAT) scan? Possibly, but that may disclose nothing too. An arthrogram of the knee, with injection of contrast material? The contrast material will easily be seen on X-ray, and the loose body's shadow may be seen moving about, yet it may well never show itself at all.

Arthroscopic surgery may be the last resort, but I remember two cases in which arthroscopy also failed to identify the loose body the first time. These movable fragments can be small enough to "hide" in several spots inside the knee, even during exploration of the joint. During arthroscopic surgery, fluid runs continuously into and out of the joint, and the loose fragment may float up, down, around, and behind the scope's tip end, never revealing itself. Most of the time, however, with patience on the surgeon's part, the loose body is found.

As for those two cases of mine, thinking ahead, I told those folks that I might not find the loose body the first time around. When I didn't, I gave each one a long piece of rubber tubing, explaining to them that if and when they felt the loose body just above the kneecap, they should wrap the rubber tube around the knee below that spot and call me right away. With the rubber tubing still in place, I could then arthroscope the area above the kneecap and remove the loose body. The technique worked—the tubing prevented the fragment from falling back into the joint and let me locate and remove it—but I believe I was just lucky in having two very observant patients.

Medial Synovial or Plica

Before arthroscopic surgery came into use, the *medial synovial plica* [PLY-ca], latin for *fold*, was entirely unknown. Only with arthroscopic techniques did we discover this lesion and recognize that it could be the source of pain. Synovial plicae are membranes that separate the knee into compartments during fetal development, normally diminishing in size between the third and six months of fetal life, and most eventually disappear. They are usually found on the medial or inside aspect of the knee, but I have seen an occasional lateral case. In children and adults, they exist as ridges of tissue or shelves. In some folks, however, the synovial plica is more prominent and prone to irritation as it glides over an edge of the medial femoral condyle (Fig. 59). There may be a crunching sound (crepitus) about the kneecap, *chondromalacia* (discussed below), which fools the surgeon into believing patellar (knee cap) disease is the cause of pain. The plica's symptoms can often imitate those of a torn medial meniscus. If all other common diagnoses are excluded during the arthroscopic examination, the orthopaedist may consider excising this piece of synovium.

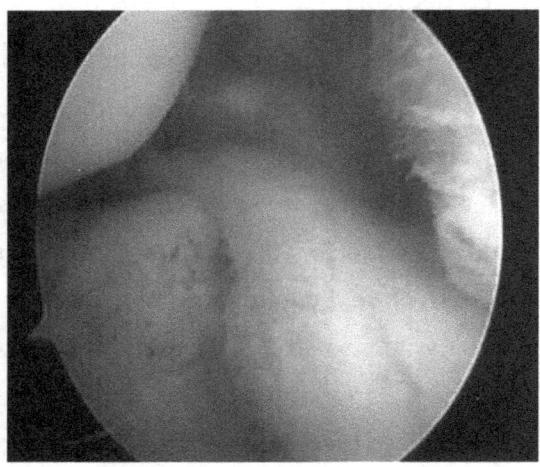

Fig. 59: Note how the white shelf of tissue (middle and right of photo) is compressed and elevated by the femoral condyle (bone) below

Iliotibial Band Syndrome

Iliotibial [illy-oh-TIB-ee-al] *band syndrome* is an inflammation and irritation at the lower outside end of the iliotibial tendon, a very long band connecting the part of the pelvis called the *ilium* [ILLY-um] to the tibia. A small bursa lies between this band and the lower, outer end of the femur close to the knee, and when an athlete runs a great deal, the continual rubbing of this band may irritate and inflame the bursa. Yes, it's our old friend bursitis causing pain again.

If an examination reveals pinpoint tenderness over the bursa as well as a tight iliotibial band, the diagnosis is clear. The pain will be on the outside of the knee, about three fingerbreadths above the lateral joint line. Your doctor will prescribe a specific passive exercise program aimed at stretching the band. The exercises usually relieve the symptoms. To avoid further tightening of the band, the exercises should be continued well after the pain is gone. No surgery is indicated with this condition.

Quadriceps Tendinitis and Rupture

Quadriceps tendinitis [QUAD-dra-ceps ten-din-NIGH-tus] is an inflammation of the quadriceps tendon, a short, wide tendon that connects the large thigh muscle—the quadriceps—to the top of the kneecap or patella. The quadriceps muscle is responsible for extending the knee from a flexed position. When this tendon becomes inflamed, it causes pain directly over the upper patella, a process similar to rotator cuff and tendon problems of the elbow. The characteristic finding is an exquisitely tender area at the point where the tendon attaches to the patella, with increased pain on pressure when the quadriceps muscle contracts. Conventional treatments are usually successful, coupled with elimination of any knee exercise that may have contributed to the disorder.

This is one situation that is definitely not appropriate for cortisone injection. While I often gave injections around or over tendons, I never injected a tendon directly as studies have shown that cortisone may weaken tendons. An inflamed tendon is already at greater risk of weakness, and even after the inflammation subsides and the tendon heals, the tendon may be weak. Injecting cortisone into it may cause further weakness and degeneration. For that reason, before a physician gives you or your family member a cortisone injection, you should always ask, "Are you injecting cortisone directly in a tendon?" Make sure the answer is no before you agree to the injection.

We know that the quadriceps tendon can weaken just like any other tendon, and it can also progress to a partial tear or a complete rupture, even without specific injury.

An elderly patient of mine who was drinking his coffee and reading the paper on Sunday morning felt so well that he jumped up from his chair to show his wife just how good he felt. When his feet hit the floor, both quadriceps tendons ruptured. I operated on him the next day, and it took him quite awhile to recover from his injury. Sad to say, he never felt quite as well again.

Pre-patellar Bursitis

Pre-patellar bursitis is, as you might suppose, an inflammation of the pre-patellar bursa, another large bursa that lies directly over the kneecap and enables skin and soft tissue to glide over the kneecap, similar to what happens in the elbow with the olecranon bursa. It, too, can become irritated, fill with fluid, and swell from trauma, gout, rheumatoid arthritis, or unknown causes. Some of this fluid may clot into small fibrous clumps called *rice bodies*, the same process that can occur in the elbow. An examiner may be able to feel these bodies slide around under finger pressure.

Drawing off the fluid for examination may be helpful in diagnosing gout, a condition known as pseudo-gout, or a bacterial infection. Sometimes, this fluid is yellow or cloudy, but tests may not yield a diagnosis. After the fluid is drawn off, a compressive bandage may help to keep more fluid from accumulating; however, it often recurs. Ultimately, if the bursitis persists with a tense fluid collection, the skin over the patella may thin out, a chronic infection may set in, or fluid may drain through a small skin opening. In these cases, the only option is surgery to remove the offending bursa surgically. Fortunately, a new bursa will grow in its place.

I have had experience with a similar condition in my own knee that I call *fibrous scarring of the pre-patellar bursa*. With this condition, the bursa scars in one small area, usually over the patella, where daily activities easily compress it. Pressing on this tiny spot causes sharp pain, but without compression, there is no pain. Slowly rubbing or sliding a finger over the bursa at the point indicated by the patient should allow the physician to identify the affected area. An injection of anesthetic and cortisone into the tender area may eliminate the pain by spreading the fibrous scar or releasing some of its adhesions as it did for me.

Patellar Subluxation or Dislocation

Patellar subluxation is a temporary partial dislocation of the kneecap from its normal position in the shallow groove on the lower front end of the femur. Episodes of subluxation can occur at any time, usually when the knee is slightly bent and the person pivots or twists toward the opposite side. The quadriceps muscle contracts, and if the groove is particularly shallow, especially in a person who has a knock-kneed stance, the patella may slide out to the lateral side. The body's immediate reflex will be to relax the quadriceps, and the knee gives way. By then, correction of the knock-kneed or twisted position can cause the kneecap to return to its normal position and brought on a second contraction of the quadriceps to keep the knee from collapsing completely. Should this second contraction be delayed or not happen at all, the person may fall. Usually, a subluxation will not damage ligaments, but each repeated episode stretches them, especially if episodes are a regular occurrence. With the subsequent loosening of the ligaments, the kneecap is more easily subluxed.

A *dislocated patella* (Fig. 60) will stay out of place, locked out over the outside portion of the femur, and can be replaced only by manipulation, usually with the patient slowly straightening the knee and allowing the patella to slide back to its original position. There are many theories as to why such a dislocation occurs. Some physicians attribute it to overdevelopment of the outer thigh muscles. Others believe it happens because the groove in which the patella rides is too shallow or flat. Still others, including me, believe a developmental knock-knee tendency allows the kneecap to slide out to the side from the force of a quadriceps contraction. A high percentage of patellar dislocations occur in women, which makes sense given that women have a wider pelvis than men, separating the upper femurs ends at the pelvis more and inclining women's knees more toward a knock-kneed stance.

Dislocations of the patella always have more drastic results than subluxation as it partially or fully ruptures the medial ligaments of the patella. Standard treatment for a first episode of patellar dislocation has always been manipulation of the kneecap back into correct position and three weeks of immobilization, followed by gradual mobilization with therapy. Being less than enthusiastic about this program myself, whenever anyone with a recent dislocation consulted me, I advised arthroscopic repair of the medial ligaments, followed by a short period of immobilization. First time ruptures of these ligaments often leaves fibers of the ligaments in different planes on both sides of the rupture. If left alone and simply immobilized, these ligaments could heal loosely or too tight. I believed performing an end-to-end repair of the ligaments, aided by the arthroscope, ensures a more nearly anatomic result.

Anyone suffering repeated episodes of subluxation or dislocation should be offered the remedy of surgery. Techniques include lateral release of soft tissue, tightening techniques, and others that reposition soft tissue and bone. The challenge in all these operations is getting the tension of the repair just right so the patella won't be too loose or too tight. While orthopaedists are rarely called on to do such surgery, the surgeon's judgment and experience will guide him in obtaining the correct tension and position of the patella and its ligaments.

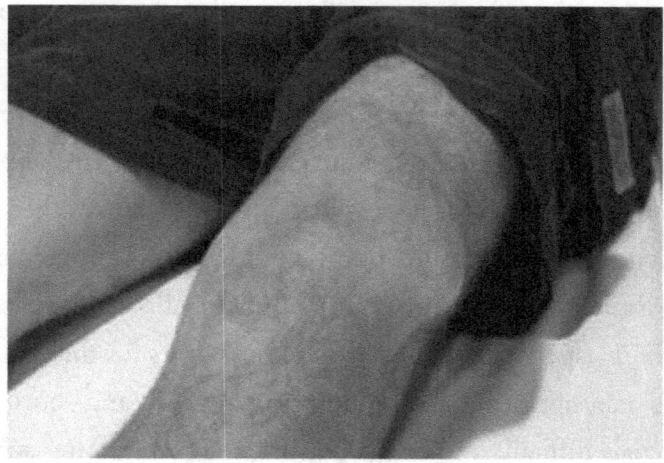

Fig. 60: Dislocated patella. Note the kneecap displaced and extending laterally from the knee
www.fightimes.com

Patellar Tendinitis and Patellar Tendon Rupture

Patellar tendinitis and *patellar tendon rupture* are still more instances of the inflammatory processes we discussed above. The condition is sometimes known as *jumper's knee*, as it often occurs in athletes who jump repetitively. In this case, the bottom of the patella where the tendon originates will be exquisitely tender and painful.

The same caution about treatment applies here: never let anyone inject this tendon. The usual treatments may help. A patellar tendon brace, a *Chopat strap*, that presses snugly against the tendon when the knee is extended may also help. Usually, these treatments and a measure of time will relieve the symptoms, although some patients may never improve, especially young athletes.

In my experience, surgical removal of the small, inflamed, and degenerated portion of tendon just to the outside of the midline of the tendon's patellar attachment often eliminated the pain. An MRI study may reveal this area of degeneration. Unfortunately, not all my cases improved with surgery, and several patients endured prolonged rehabilitation before they improved. Results were good to excellent, however, in 75–80 percent of my cases.

The patellar tendon, like other tendons, can rupture. A careful history from a patient who suffered this injury may disclose that the patient had a tender and painful area over the lower aspect of the kneecap before the rupture occurred. Acute rupture of this tendon calls for immediate surgical attention. Rather than rupturing in its middle, this tendon usually pulls off the inferior aspect of the patella, and if one waits for the acute injury to heal rather than operating, the tendon may contract and shorten, making eventual repair difficult and compromising the result. After such surgery, rehabilitation can take as long as a year before the patient regains a full range of motion and strength.

Patellar Chondromalacia

Patellar chondromalacia [KON-dro-ma-LAY-shi-a] is a degenerative condition of the cartilage that covers the back of the patella (*chondro-* refers to the hyaline cartilage covering a bone, and *-malacia* means "damage to"). More specifically, changes in the deepest layers of cartilage cause blistering and fragmentation of the cartilage that covers the back surface of the kneecap (Fig. 61), which ordinarily glides over the lower end of the femur in the knee joint. The condition is also known as *runner's knee*, as it happens to many athletes who run long distances although I'm not convinced that running is the cause of this condition since many of those folks I treated were not runners. It seems to be a localized fragmentation of the hyaline cartilage that does not specifically progress to *patello-femoral arthritis*, a painful condition affecting both surfaces of the patella and its articulation with the femur in the knee.

Patellar chondromalacia does not necessarily cause pain. This is important. In fact, most folks I've seen who demonstrate crepitus—those characteristic crunching and snapping sounds as the kneecap rides irregularly over the femur—have no pain. Their pain is actually caused by some other condition within or about the knee. A physician who detects this crepitus may reach the false conclusion that chondromalacia is causing the symptoms, yet in many cases, nothing is further from the truth. I believe chondromalacia is one of the most frequently mistaken diagnoses in orthopaedics, and a careful physician must rule out all other possible common knee problems before saddling someone with this diagnosis.

I say this for several reasons. Many young people complain of crunching in their knees, especially when going downstairs, yet have no pain. If there truly were as many cases of chondromalacia as are diagnosed, we should see far more of it than we do as our patients age. In addition, a high percentage of folks who have crepitus eventually improve without surgery, going on with their lives pain-free but with persistent crepitus.

Does chondromalacia ever cause pain? Yes. In some cases, the fragmented cartilage flakes off into the knee joint, causing a reactive inflammation of the synovium, the membrane encasing the joint. I have seen irritation and thickening of the synovium around the patella caused by bits and pieces of cartilage lodged within it, so in these cases, chondromalacia did seem to contribute to the pain. *Coblation* (a procedure using heat to smooth the irregular surface) of the irregular cartilage reduces the chances that more fragments will break loose and fall into the joint. Before this advancement was available, we used to shave the back of the patella to rid it of these loose fragments, but the visible end results were never even and smooth as that obtained by coblation. Before arthroscopy was available, we would actually trim the irregular changes on the kneecap's undersurface with a knife. Today's techniques are more perfected for this disease processes, and the results are so much better.

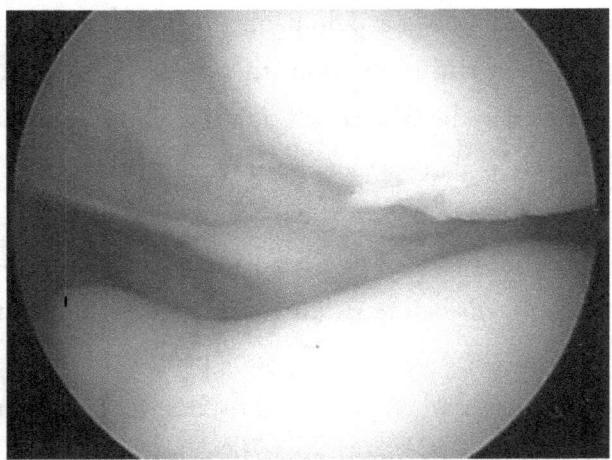

Fig. 61: Patellar chondromalacia. Note the fragmenting piece hanging off the undersurface of the kneecap

Pes Anserine Bursitis

Still another bursa in the area of the knee, the *pes anserine* (AN-sir-een) *bursa* can become irritated and cause symptoms. It takes its name from the Latin meaning "goose foot" because of its webbed appearance. This bursa lies beneath two conjoining tendons that connect parts of the hamstring muscles to the top of the inside portion of the upper tibia and serves to help the tendons glide over the tibia. In the absence of any other disorder, the pes anserine bursa can become inflamed—bursitis—to cause pain just below the middle front of the knee always below the joint line. If this bursitis is not recognized, the physician may attribute the pain to the medial meniscus. Pinpoint pressure over this bursa will reproduce the pain, however, and a local injection of anesthetic and cortisone usually eliminates the symptoms. No surgery is required for this condition.

Medial Collateral Ligament Bursitis

Earlier, we discussed the medial collateral ligament (MCL). It, too, is associated with a bursa, the *medial collateral ligament bursa*, which lies between the bottom end of the MCL and its attachment to the tibia. Like most other bursae, this one can also become locally inflamed. If not pinpointed on exam, this pain can also be mistaken for pain from the medial meniscus, and the wrong remedy applied.

Before rushing into any diagnosis of an orthopaedic condition, especially having to do with the knee, a physician will carry out a comprehensive physical examination. Because many of the structures we've been discussing lie very close together, it will be up to the physician to distinguish the pain pattern of one from some other condition. A local anesthetic/steroid injection will also usually eliminate the symptoms of an MCL bursitis.

By now, you may be thinking I gave a great many injections when I was in practice. It's true. I did, but many of them were aids in making the correct diagnosis. If the local anesthetic knocked out the patient's pain entirely, I knew I had the proper diagnosis, and rather than giving two injections, I added the refined steroid with the anesthetic injection to treat the problem. Having carried out a comprehensive history and physical exam, I was always relatively certain of the diagnosis; therefore, I did not inject indiscriminately. Not only is this technique an excellent diagnostic aid, but the patient is extremely grateful for instant relief of the pain and for my saving them time and money by eliminating the need for multiple visits.

Making the exact diagnosis is the most important part of the practice of medicine. As some say, this is an art. Because many pains are so closely related, the doctor faces the challenge of identifying the offending body part, and in many cases, I found an injection of a local anesthetic to be the quickest and cheapest way to find out what I needed to know.

Anterior Fat Pad Syndrome

The knee joint contains a triangular fat pad behind the patellar tendon (Fig.51), the pad being tethered to the anterior aspects of the anterior cruciate and femoral notch by a short ligament (the *ligamentum mucosa*). I was often asked to see children from ages twelve to seventeen who complained of pain on the front of the knee when active, many having been previously diagnosed with patellar chondromalacia or a torn lateral meniscus. Some, but certainly not all, did have some degree of chondromalacia but not enough to treat, and none had a torn meniscus. If they stopped whatever activity caused the pain, it subsided, only to return with more activity.

I thought the tethering ligament might be part of the problem. On examination of most knees, full extension of the knee pushes the fat pad forward, creating a bulge to the lateral aspect of the patellar tendon. In these youngsters, if I pressed on this soft area while the knee was bent and maintained that pressure as they fully straightened the knee, they complained of the same pain. I was able to confirm my theory by arthroscoping their knees and simply snipping this short tethering ligament, with a high percentage of success.

Osgood-Schlatter's Disease

Osgood-Schlatter's Disease, named for the two men who first described it, is another condition I have suffered as a boy. Interestingly, this disease was described by these two men—one English and the other German—without the benefit of either man knowing the other.

The section of bone where the patellar tendon attaches to the tibia (the *tibial tuberosity*) becomes inflamed through either overuse or some loss of blood supply, and its bony attachment fragments. A person affected by the disorder will complain of pain, often in both knees, directly over the tibial tuberosity. The pain can be quite debilitating, especially in running and contact sports. For someone with Osgood-Schlatter's disease, a fall to the knees can bring on severe acute pain that gradually eases over a period of ten to fifteen minutes. Osgood-Schlatter's disease occurs most often in children, mainly growing boys ages ten to sixteen who run and jump a lot as those activities put a much greater strain on the patellar tendon than other activities do.

The disorder begins with persistent inflammation and irritation of the periosteum, the outer covering layer of bone that generates new bone cells. During healing periods, as new bone is laid down, the tibial tuberosity becomes enlarged. When youngsters stop growing and the tendons gain strength, the disorder clears up. Tincture of time, kneepads with cutouts for the enlarged area, ibuprofen, and rest may help, but ultimately, the condition stops once the boy finishes growing. There is no place here for cortisone injections.

During my years in practice, I saw several adults who had had Osgood-Schlatter's disease and were still bothered by a loose bone fragment in the knee as a result of the process. Removing this loose fibrous or bony material was usually all that was necessary for complete relief.

Osteochondritis Dissecans (OCD)

The disorder's name describes it: inflammation and fragmentation of hyaline cartilage over bone. *Osteochondritis* [oss-tee-oh-kon-DRY-tis] *dissecans* [DISS-ek-cans] generally happens in one of the femoral condyles, the large knoblike structures at the lower end of the femur. OCD affects adults up to age fifty, and the juvenile form (JOCD) affects children nine years old and up (Fig 62). While no one is certain what causes OCD, physicians have speculated that repetitive activities, a mechanical disruption of blood flow to bone, or both cause part of the end of the bone to die, a condition I discussed in the femoral head, *avascular necrosis*.

In the first stage of this condition, part of the bone dies though the overlying hyaline cartilage, which derives nourishment from the synovial fluid rather than from blood, does not. The small dead bone fragment can then work loose under its intact cartilage cover. In the next stage, the overlying cartilage splits, leaving both bone and cartilage partly loose. In the last stage of the disease, the cartilage and bone fragment together fall into the joint (Fig. 62).

In a youngster with JOCD, rest of the affected knee and avoidance of all sports for at least ten months, sometimes as long as eighteen months, will usually heal the knee. Repeated bone scans may indicate the progress of healing; however, some cases do not heal and go on to become adult OCD.

Early diagnosis is the key. Unfortunately, the initial symptoms may be too mild for a patient to seek medical advice. Even when the child is brought for evaluation, the history is generally vague, and the physical exam is normal. X-rays may appear to be normal in the early stages. Nevertheless, the physician must be very much aware of this disease process and review periodic X-rays for any minute bone change on the lower end of the femur. As time passes, knee pain may increase, sometimes until the youngster is unable to bear weight fully on that knee and may complain of snapping sensations and the knee giving way. While an MRI study is probably the best way to diagnose the disease, a bone scan may also be useful.

Before proper treatment begins, the patient and his family must be educated as to its possible progression and consequences. Surgery is usually the only effective treatment for OCD. If only bone is damaged, with the overlying cartilage intact, drilling the bone to promote bone healing through a new blood supply with or without small fixation devices may be successful. If the bone and cartilage fragments are partially loose or have fallen off, the same procedure may be tried, first peeling back the loose piece and shaving the bony base to promote new bleeding, then pinning the fragments back in place (Fig. 63).

For a fragment on the weight-bearing end of the bone, this procedure should certainly be tried even though the fragment and the base from which it came may no longer be a good fit. Trimming the fragment and sculpting the base to match is extremely difficult and time-consuming. Some surgeons repair the defect using the patient's own bone and cartilage from elsewhere in the knee (an autograft), while others use tissue from bone and cartilage banks (an allograft).

In a newer technique, *autologous* [aw-TALL-oh-gus] *chondrocyte* [KON-dro-sight] *implantation*, cartilage cells from the patient, are grown in the lab and inserted into the OCD defect to encourage growth of new hyaline cartilage. This approach requires two operations, the first to obtain the patient's cells for the laboratory to culture, the second to introduce the new cells into the bony defect and cover them with the patient's own tissue. This operation is also very time-consuming and must be meticulously performed. Time will tell if this technique has high success.

Ultimately, if all else fails, the fragment may simply have to be removed.

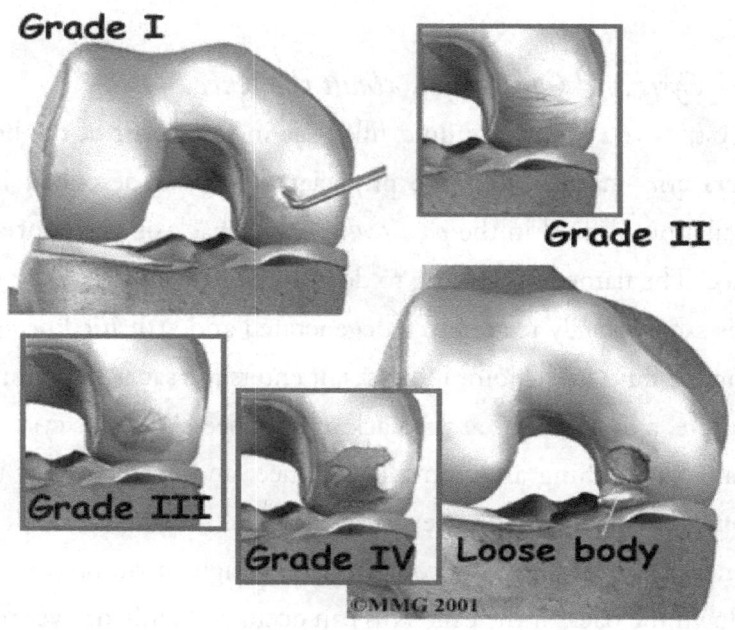

Fig. 62: Grades of OCD:
1. Loose bone under intact cartilage. 2. Cartilage now being affected.
3. Bone and cartilage loose but not separated.
4. Bone and cartilage separated and fallen into joint, forming a loose body.
Image courtesy of Medical Multimedia Group, LLC,
www.eOrthopod.com

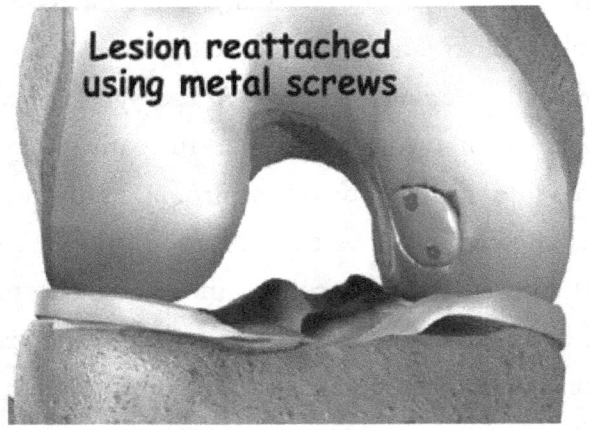

Fig. 63: Bone and cartilage fragment trimmed and pinned into its original base
Image courtesy of Medical Multimedia Group, LLC, www.eOrthopod.com

Baker's Cysts and Other Cysts about the Knee

A cyst, as you know, is a fluid-filled sac in some part of the body, and a *Baker's cyst*—named after the physician who first described it—is an accumulation of fluid in the *popliteal space*, or back or posterior aspect of the knee. The name has nothing to do with being a baker!

This sac is usually related to a degenerated and arthritic knee joint. As the amount fluid in the joint increases, it enters the sac. After enough fluid pools there, a bulge forms at the back of the knee. A Baker's cyst is usually a signal of something amiss inside the knee, and correction of the knee problem will usually reduce the size of the cyst.

Sometimes, such a cyst becomes large enough to rupture, forcing the fluid down the back of the calf. This can occur suddenly or over time. The pain in an acute case may be similar to the pain of *thrombophlebitis* [thrombo-fla-BITE-tiss], a deep vein inflammation with a blood clot formation. Because such a blood clot can migrate to the lung, sometimes with fatal consequences, many physicians will hasten to prescribe blood-thinning medication for someone who may simply have a ruptured Baker's cyst. If there is any question about the diagnosis, an ultrasound study or *Doppler examination* should settle the matter, as it will be positive for clots and negative for a ruptured cyst.

The back of the knee contains other bursal cysts unrelated to the joint and usually present long before the patient recognizes their existence. While they cause no pain or harm to the patient, the physician may draw off the fluid from them. Surgery to remove them or a true Baker's cyst is rarely indicated.

Osteoarthritis of the Knee

Osteoarthritis of the knee, an uneven deterioration of the bone ends at the joint, can come about through injury, internal derangements of the knee described above, rheumatoid arthritis, gout, pseudo-gout, bacterial infection, and other causes. As a rule, however, folks with osteoarthritis of the knee have no such history. Many will have some fluid in the knee, a joint that remains bent to some degree (called a *flexion contracture*), and be unable to straighten the knee entirely because of bony deformity and tight ligaments. Patient may present with knock-kneed or bowlegged deformities. Some folks can straighten the knee but bend it only so far. Several areas of the knee may be tender. Nearly everyone with systematic osteoarthritic knees will limp, and some may need a cane or a crutch when they walk. Others may have only intermittent knee pain and swelling and be able to walk unassisted.

X-ray examination of an osteoarthritic knee will show narrowing of one or both compartments in the knee. Normally, there is a space between the bones on X-ray. This space is the area of the hyaline cartilage on the end of the femur and tibia I have already discussed. This cartilage does not show up on X-ray, so only a space is visible between the bones. When the cartilage is fragmented and wears away, the space often narrows so much that we see bone on bone on X-ray, meaning there is absolutely no more cartilage covering on either the femur or the tibia. Bone spurs (*osteophytes*) will be seen on the femoral condyles, the knob-like protrusions on the edges of the femur. An MRI evaluation will show severe loss of hyaline cartilage and deformity of the condyles.

Many forms of osteoarthritis exist. The physician's experience with the disorder dictates the treatment. All the conservative treatments and forms of therapy we've mentioned for other conditions may be used, and removing fluid from the knee using a needle and syringe, along with injection of local anesthetic and refined steroid, may reduce the inflammation and pain.

Some folks believe the oral compound *glucosamine with chrondroitin sulfate* helps to reduce osteoarthritic symptoms. Injections of *visco-supplements*, a synthetic fluid to supplement the knee's natural synovial fluid, have also provided some temporary relief of pain and improved the joint's ability to withstand stresses of daily activities. In my experience, however, glucosamine, chondroitin, and visco-supplements have all failed to produce good long-term results in the majority of patients. Some patients swear by them and others swear at them. They may be worth trying, but I believe that eventually some better forms of therapy will be developed.

You may have seen "before and after" X-rays of knees in advertisements for certain medications in which one or the other of these treatments is said to have "revived" the joint space. A closer look at these X-rays will reveal the angle of the X-ray beam and the knee in the "after" film to be different from the "before" film, supposedly showing that the joint space has "opened up." These photographs have failed to convince me that these drugs work. I know of very few peer review studies—research from respected orthopaedists and reviewed by other orthopaedists—that report high rates of success from either therapy. Even if successful results were reported, I believe the improvement would be only temporary.

If you could actually see the severe changes in a knee at arthroscopy, you would understand how I just can't see how a medication—oral or injectable—can reverse these changes. There will always be disagreement, of course, and my position will surely spawn some criticism, but it's the way I see it.

Once all conservative management has been exhausted, and the patient's pain and lifestyle limitations are severe enough, surgery may be in order. It's the surgeon's responsibility to inform the patient fully of all its potential consequences and complications.

Two different operations may be considered. One, an arthroscopic procedure, is essentially a "housecleaning" of the joint. The surgeon washes out all loose material, trims, and removes irregular pieces of hyaline cartilage and menisci, and heat treats areas of synovitis by coblation. In my practice, I saw some patients with arthritic joints whose pain seemed to be caused only by a tear of a meniscus—a loose piece that periodically got trapped between the bone ends. Arthroscopic removal of the meniscus fragment gave these patients much relief for many years, and while some eventually needed total knee replacement, others never did. Since I have osteoarthritic knees and degenerative menisci in both, I believe I would have an arthroscopic procedure to trim my lateral meniscus and wash out my knee before undergoing a total knee replacement.

The other alternative for a severely deteriorated knee joint is the open procedure called a *total knee arthroplasty* (TKA), in which the surgeon removes the lower end of the femur and replaces it with composite metal condyles and removes the upper end of the tibia and replaces it with a plastic substitute. In rare cases, a *hemiarthroplasty* will suffice, replacing only half of the joint.

Before entertaining the idea of a TKA operation, particularly in younger patients, some surgeons believe an osteotomy of the tibia or the femur— cutting and setting a bone at a different angle to alter the forces placed on the arthritic knee—may be beneficial. Many of these procedures have been successful, but in cases that do not improve, the angle change can make the TKA a more technically difficult operation. I don't know how many surgeons use this technique routinely although as more and more young patients are seen for osteoarthritis, the procedure is becoming more acceptable.

The TKA is a definitive procedure. Once bone is removed and replaced with prosthetic devices, there's no going back. That's why I would suggest an arthroscopic procedure as a first line of operative defense.

The rehabilitation after a TKA is intense. Immediately after the operation, most knees are placed in a CPM (*constant passive motion*) machine. Constant motion of the knee during the immediate postoperative period will decrease the likelihood of dense adhesions that will subsequently chip away at the patient's ability to obtain good functional motion. The machine is initially set at full extension and mild flexion, and the flexion angle is increased as the patient's pain allows. Patients must be instructed in the use of the machine because they often are sent home with such a machine to continue their therapy. As with the ACL surgeries, I encouraged my folks to work very hard on actively extending their knees during this most important period. Often, they become obsessed with regaining flexion of their knee and do not realize that they are not fully extending the knee. If full extension is not obtained, the patient will walk with a limp, the extremity effectively being shorter than the opposite side. The screw home mechanism will be lost, and the strength of the quadriceps muscle will be compromised.

Postoperative follow-up in the doctor's office should be quite often in the first six weeks. In that way, the surgeon can observe any problems with the wound, infectious processes, and loss of function. Physical therapy is almost always necessary to help the patient over some tough times. A patient will rarely be able to rehabilitate himself without some sort of formal help.

CHAPTER 15
THE TIBIA

Shin Splints

Most people who have run for exercise or trained for sports necessitating a good deal of running have had shin splints or *periostitis* [perry-os-TIE-tis], an inflammation of the outer covering, the *periosteum*, of the tibia that is the major bone of the lower leg. The condition usually appears the day of or the day after an intensive running stint, manifesting as tenderness along the inside front or anterior aspect of the lower leg. It may disappear quickly but return with the next run. Rarely is there any associated swelling.

Its cause is thought to be repetitive traction on the lining of the tibia at the spot where the *tibialis posterior* muscle originates. As a rule, I found that affected patients had a moderately to severely *pronated* [PRO-nate-ed] *foot* (Fig. 64), with a relatively flattened arch and bearing weight mostly on the inside of the foot. Because the tendon of the tibialis posterior muscle rides along the inside of the ankle to the middle sole of the foot, the muscle is overstretched and repetitively pulls at its origin on the tibia and its periosteum. This traction produces an inflammatory reaction and the pain of shin splints.

Correction of the pronation by means of orthotics and shock-absorbing insoles (a short course of anti-inflammatory medication) and taping of the ankle to hold in the body's natural heat and prevent pronation should help to alleviate the shin splints. If the person must or wants to continue to run, an ongoing exercise program to stretch the calf muscle, especially the tibialis posterior, should be prescribed.

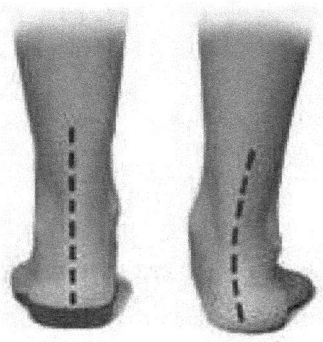

Fig. 64: Pronated foot on the right corrected by orthotic on the left
www.sportsinjuryclinic.net

Posterior Compartment Syndrome

The deep calf muscles of the back of the lower leg are enclosed in a sheath known as the posterior compartment of the tibia. When one of these muscles becomes too swollen for the sheath, causing pain, the condition is known as a *compartment syndrome*. Compartment syndromes can be acute or chronic. The cause is usually either an injury to the muscle from overuse, causing the muscle to swell within its confines and never get a chance to fully recover over time, or an acute impact or muscle tear that causes bleeding and sudden swelling within the compartment. A compartment syndrome can also occur in the anterior compartment where the *anterior tibialis* muscle resides. When present, it can masquerade as shin splints, but it is found on the outer front side of the tibia rather than the inner.

A chronic compartment syndrome is usually the result of overuse of these muscles for a considerable period of time, as, for example, with too frequent or too lengthy running. The pressure within the muscle compartment never really returns to normal, and continued running tends to add to it, causing the muscle to bulge against its lining, the *fascia* [FASH-yah] that, in turn, causes a deep aching pain. This pain may disappear with cessation of activity only to return soon after the next bout of exercise.

Acute compartment syndromes are usually caused by a blow to the calf or a severe muscle tear that initiates bleeding within the muscle and the lining. The swelling continues because of the bleeding, increasing the pressure within the muscle quickly. The diagnosis of an acute compartment syndrome is easily made on the basis of a swollen and hard, tender calf muscle. Because the pressure can build so quickly in these deep muscles and cause death of the muscle, the physician should be familiar with the five *P*'s that are danger signs: pain, pallor (loss of normal color) of the foot, paresthesia (numbness and tingling), paralysis, and pulseless (reduced or no pulse) in the ankle or foot. These may be signs that the soft tissues have suffered extensive and irreversible injuries, so their presence constitutes an orthopaedic emergency. A *fasciotomy* [FAS-she-ot-toe-me]—a surgical operation to decompress these muscles—is absolutely necessary at this point.

Intramuscular pressure can be measured with needlelike structures—transducers connected to catheters—placed within the compartments of the calf. In an acute compartment syndrome, typical pressures at rest range from 30–45 mm of mercury. Because time is the enemy with this condition, however, I would be greatly concerned if the physician wasted valuable minutes measuring and documenting pressures. Waiting for these studies can mean muscle death and permanent injury. I believe that when a strong possibility of acute compartment syndrome exists, the physician should forgo measuring pressures, inform the patient of the gravity of the situation and, with the patient's consent, carry out an immediate decompression.

On the other hand, intramuscular or intra-compartmental pressure measurements are necessary to confirm the diagnosis of a chronic compartment syndrome. In chronic compartment syndrome, resting intra-compartmental pressures greater than 15 mm of mercury or a pressure greater than 30 mm of mercury with exertion are generally considered elevated. In this case, if measurements indicate a constant elevation of pressure, especially with activity, the surgeon should offer the patient an elective decompression (fasciotomy) of the muscles to relieve the pain.

Achilles Tendinitis and Rupture

By now, you know that almost all tendons can suffer some idiopathic loss of blood supply, the body reacting with an inflammatory response in an attempt to heal the tendon. We've seen this in the rotator cuff, the elbow, and the tendons about the wrist, hand, and knee. The same is true of the Achilles' [ah-KILL-eez] tendon, the tendon of the *gastrocnemius* [gas-trock-NEE-me-us], the largest calf muscle.

Medicine has assigned strange names to many parts of the body, most of them taken from the Latin language. This tendon's name comes from the Greek story of the mythological hero, Achilles, who died of a poisoned arrow wound in the heel. Until so wounded, he had been invulnerable. When he was young, his mother had dipped him in the River Styx whose waters supposedly protected against injury and death. As she immersed him, however, she kept her grip on his heel that failed to receive the protection.

The Achilles tendon extends from the calf muscle down behind the ankle and attaches to the upper back of the heel bone, the *calcaneus* [kal-KANE-ee-us] or also known as the *os calcis* [oss -KAL-sis]. If you've heard of someone's having a torn Achilles tendon, this is the structure that ruptured. Sometimes, when a degenerative process affects the Achilles tendon, the person may never feel the initial insult but will, over a period of time, become aware of an insidious aching or tenderness in the tendon's midsection, soon followed by a tender swelling that eventually becomes apparent to the eye. At this stage of inflammation or tendinitis, he or she may not realize what's happening, only that something seems different.

If the person seeks medical attention while the tendon is inflamed but has not pulled away from its attachment, the approach to treatment will be extremely important. The physician must explain how serious a full rupture of this tendon would be, stressing the need to avoid any activity that may cause such a rupture. So long as the tendon is diseased, the person must—at all costs—avoid any activity that requires a quick or sudden push off the foot. All jumping and landing on the foot in ordinary daily activities, let alone sports, must also be avoided. Anti-inflammatory medication, heat, ultrasound, and electrical stimulation may reduce the pain but can't be counted on to reduce the time needed for healing.

A patient appeared in my office years ago with the classic signs of Achilles tendinitis. When I told him the tendon could rupture if he continued to play squash, he seemed to understand and, with time and some therapy, seemed to improve. But then, despite my continued emphasis on the need to avoid playing squash until all was well, he played anyway and ruptured the tendon, pulling it off the heel bone. The final outcome was far from perfect, necessitating several surgeries and lengthy periods of immobilization.

So long as any tendinitis persists, the tendon remains weak, especially its central portion. Even though it feels thicker and may no longer be tender, its midsection may have lost all tendinous continuity. An MRI evaluation should be done to evaluate the healing of this inflammatory reaction, especially in professional athletes. It's not uncommon to see professional athletes helped off the field with a ruptured Achilles tendon.

The area of weakness in the unguarded tendon will finally give way, caused by an acute stretching of the tendon or contraction of the calf muscle. The tendon may rupture in any of three areas: at its musculotendinous junction with the calf muscle, at its midsection, or at the heel bone. Most ruptures happen at the middle of the tendon. The symptoms are acute pain and inability to push the foot downward (*plantar flexion*) or walk on one's toes.

Most of these midsection ruptures require an operation using one of multiple techniques. The surgeon will incise the healthy sheath surrounding the rupture in order to observe the rupture and then use sutures to reconnect the torn parts. Because the suturing of these tendon results in a thicker tendon mass, the surrounding sheath, subcutaneous tissue, and the skin incision can be a bit difficult to close without some lingering tension.

The foot and ankle must be immobilized for some length of time, depending on the individual case, with gradual motion begun while still protecting the repair. As a rule, three months of protection without bearing weight will be needed, followed by another six months of careful exercising to regain full range of motion. All patients must be told emphatically to avoid quick plantar flexion of the foot, as the tendon may not be fully healed for a year. Each surgeon has his own rehabilitation program, and the patient should inquire as to when he will be fully ambulatory and can return to sports.

Complications of this surgery include wound healing, infection, loss of motion, calf atrophy and weakness, and re-rupture. All calf muscles will atrophy as a result of the disuse and immobilization, and a permanent smaller calf muscle may result despite an intense exercise program.

While I was in the navy, I saw a soldier with an Achilles rupture in my clinic. The rupture was three weeks old. I scheduled him for surgery, but his medical doctor would not let him undergo surgery, determining from the patient's abnormal electrocardiogram that he'd recently suffered a silent heart attack.

I had just read an article by an orthopaedist who treated many Achilles tendon injuries as a prison physician. Evidently, prisoners would cut their

Achilles tendon to avoid work. They knew they would be operated on and would have an easier life in the hospital and during rehab than the other prisoners. This physician finally decided to cast the foot and ankle of these men for three months and rehab them as he would have done, if he'd operated them. No surgery! His results were quite good, rivaling those for patients he did operate on. I decided to try this technique with my patient even though his injury was three weeks old. I had no other alternative. To my surprise, he healed very well and eventually had a functional Achilles tendon.

Afterward, I decided to use this technique on all midsection and musculotendinous Achilles tendon ruptures. I operated only on the tendons that had ruptured off the bone. My theory was that the two portions of the tendon were still within their sheath, and if I immobilized them with the foot in its most plantar-flexed position, the two ends would approximate each other within their own blood clot and the sheath. There would be no surgical incision into the sheath surrounding the tendon parts, allowing for a tunnel across which the parts could oppose each other. The clot would eventually form a dense fibrous connection between the two sections just as it would if I'd operated. Every two weeks, I'd change the cast and bring the foot up a little until I removed the cast after three months. I would increase the heel size of patients' shoes or encourage them to wear cowboy boots to take tension off the repair while they were regaining full motion and calf strength. Of course, they were advised to avoid push-off and jumping. I would protect all of these repairs for a total of nine months.

With this technique, I avoided any skin problems and infections. I used this technique in over sixty tendon ruptures. All healed. Over time, I had three re-ruptured repairs. One occurred a year after repair as the patient ran to catch a bus. The other two were in noncompliant patients. One fellow went horseback riding a week after his cast was removed and jumped off his horse. The other patient proceeded to play tennis six weeks after cast removal. When asked why they didn't comply with my instructions, they both answered, "It didn't hurt, so I thought it was healed." Despite constant reminders, patients often choose to count on their own feelings and impulses. Some get away with it, and others don't.

I have seen MRI studies of "healed" Achilles tendons a year after repair, both surgical and non-surgical. Central portions of some of these tendons still showed no tendinous material. In theory, these tendons are not completely healed. All patients must understand that re-rupture of the tendon may occur even though seemingly healed even after a year.

Calcaneal Apophysitis

Calcaneal (Cal-can-knee-al) Apophysitis (A-pop-fis-sy-tis), otherwise known as Sever's disease, is found only in growing children. The back portion of the heel in these patients has a growth center known as an *apophysis* [a-POP-fiss-sis]. An apophysis is similar to an epiphysis but does not contribute to growth. The apophysis is separated from the main bone until the child finishes growing, and then the cartilage between it and becomes bone. The Achilles tendon attaches here as well. With overuse, running and jumping, the area can become inflamed, slightly swollen, and very tender and painful. Reduction of activity, ice or heat, and rest are components of treatment. The pain will disappear after the child finishes growing and the apophysis becomes a permanent part of the heel bone. No residual problems will result. Sever's disease is somewhat similar to the Osgood-Schlatter's disease of the tibia.

CHAPTER 16
THE ANKLE

The ankle or *talocrural* [tail-oh-CREW-ral] joint has multiple bony and ligamentous components. We've already discussed the tibia and the fibula, the two long bones of the lower leg. The fibula is the smaller of the two, attached to the tibia by a ligamentous structure, the *interosseous* [in-TER-os-ee-us] membrane, and ligaments at the top and bottom of the fibula. When someone walks, the fibula actually moves up and down a bit as ligaments are its only attachment to the tibia. The lower ends of both the tibia and the fibula form part of the ankle.

I like to view the ankle as an upside-down saddle joint, one side being an extension of the L-shaped lower end of the tibia or *medial malleolus* [mal-LEEL-lus]. The lower end of the fibula or *lateral malleolus* is the other side of the saddle. The malleoli (plural for *malleolus*) are those prominent roundish bones that can be seen and felt at your ankle, one on the inside and the other on the outside of the ankle. In the middle of the saddle is the third bone making up the ankle joint—the *talus,* a part of the foot.

Multiple circumferential ligaments support the ankle so it can bear the body's entire weight. On the inner side of the ankle, there is a large triangular structure, the *deltoid ligament*, which attaches the talus to the medial malleolus. The several ligaments that hold the tibia and the fibula at the ankle are known, reasonably enough, as the *tibio-fibular* [TIB-be-oh-FIB-yew-lar] *ligaments*, while the *fibulo-talar* [FIB-bew-low-TAIL-lar] *ligaments* connect the fibula and the talus on the ankle's outer side. An up and down rocking movement of the talus within the confines of the saddle gives us plantar flexion, with the foot angled downward, and dorsiflexion, with the foot angled up (Fig. 65).

Even though wonderfully constructed, the ankle joint is inherently unstable. Our heel bone, the calcaneus, sits under the talus. The calcaneus can rock inward (*inversion*) or outward (*eversion*), thereby tilting the foot to the left and right. This motion is not in the ankle but in solely in the *talocalcaneal* or *subtalar* joint (Fig. 66). So in review, the rocking up and down of the talus occurs in the ankle joint, and the tilting of the foot inward and outward is performed in the joint between the talus and heel bone, not in the ankle. Multiple perfectly placed ligaments also provide this joint with a degree of stability.

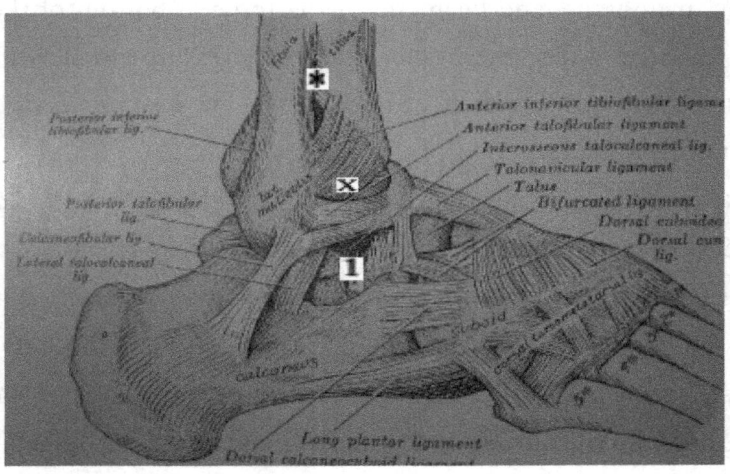

Fig. 66: Ligaments of lateral side of right ankle. Note the height of the ligaments extending up between the fibula and the tibia (x). Ligaments ruptured with high ankle sprains occur at * or higher.
Sinus tarsi (1).
Gray's Anatomy, 1966

Sprained Ankle

Why does this subtalar joint theoretically make the ankle joint unstable? As soon as person either inverts or everts the talo-calcaneal joint, undue stress forces can be transmitted through the talus, placing tension and stretching on the ligaments that hold it in the upside-down saddle. Forces on a foot tilted inward will cause tension and possible rupture of the lateral ligaments of the ankle joint, whereas forces on an outwardly tilted foot will place tension on the medial ligaments of the ankle. If either of these positions happens to be extreme, as when one "turns his ankle," the ligaments may stretch or give way, with a sprained ankle as the result.

Typically, the sprained ankle occurs after *hyper-inversion* of the foot—that is, a drastic inward turning or tilting of the foot, as when a person comes down suddenly with increased force on an already turned-in foot, thereby stressing the outside ligaments of the ankle. Such injuries are common after a jump in basketball, when players come down off-balance onto one foot. These lateral ligaments can either tear slightly at their lowest end, the injury may continue upward from the tibio-calcaneal ligaments to involve the lower tibio-fibular ligaments (Fig. 66 x) or, higher, to the upper tibio-fibular ligaments (Fig. 66 *), or even higher, to the tibio-fibular interosseous membrane. We refer to such an injury as a *high ankle sprain*. Football and basketball players, who move at high speeds and expose their feet and legs to heavy impact, will have most of the high ankle sprains. Because enormous force is required to rupture all these ligaments, an orthopaedist in private practice will, fortunately, not see many such cases.

Someone who tears the lower lateral ligaments will feel acute pain and sometimes feel or hear a pop, followed almost immediately by swelling from a blood clot or hematoma on the side of the ankle and pain with any effort to bear weight. Proper treatment is application of ice for the first twenty-four to forty-eight hours, followed by application of wet heat, elevation of the ankle above the level of one's heart to reduce swelling, rest, and avoidance of weight-bearing until the ankle is comfortable again. Some physicians will use a soft, or even a plaster, walking cast for about three weeks to allow the ligaments to heal, after which exercise is necessary to increase the joint's range of motion, stretch the healed ligaments back to their normal length, and restore strength to the muscles about the joint. Inversion stretching—turning the ankle inward—will be necessary to lengthen the healed but shortened ligaments on the outside of the ankle.

Eversion injuries, those in which the foot rotated outward, are more difficult to treat. With a fairly simple eversion injury, the medial deltoid ligament is sometimes but not always sprained. How does this happen? As the foot turns outward, the talus must also rotate outward within the saddle of the joint, twisting and stressing the fibula, pushing and rotating it outward as well. At the same time, stresses affecting the tibio-fibular ligaments on the outside of the ankle can also stretch the deltoid ligament on the medial side. Unrelenting rotation can eventually rupture ligaments higher on the outside as well as the deltoid ligament. Usually, a pure inversion injury will cause swelling laterally, and an eversion injury will cause swelling medially.

However, if the ankle is swollen on both sides, even with no broken bone, the doctor must realize he is dealing with multiple injured ankle ligaments. An X-ray may show a normal ankle, even if the ankle is totally unstable. It will be up to the physician to reconstruct the mechanism of injury by questioning the patient as to exactly what happened. Some patients remember; some won't. In any case, the ankle will be severely swollen on both sides, and the doctor, with gentle manipulation, may be able to rock the talus back and forth to identify the site of instability. A neuro-vascular exam—a careful investigation of nerves and blood vessels—is essential to make sure the ankle did not completely dislocate and then go back into place unassisted before the patient came to the hospital or the doctor's office.

The Ankle

Usually, the injury will fall somewhere between the worst-case scenario and a deltoid-ligament sprain. Appropriate treatment is as described above. Elevation above the level of the patient's heart must be emphasized and reemphasized. I always told my patients that their outcome depended solely on keeping their ankle elevated this way for at least seven days. Of course, no one wanted to hear this, and many resisted mightily, but I found it to be the best treatment without a doubt.

If the swelling goes down significantly in three to five days, all is well and good, and the patient can begin partial to full weight-bearing, but if the swelling persists, a longer period of elevation will be necessary. You see, it's the blood that escaped from the ruptured tissues that made the ankle swell in the first place, and in time, this blood will clot and turn to fibrous tissue and finally—you guessed it—to scar tissue. This limits the ankle's motion and causes discomfort and pain for a long time afterward. That was the basis for my rule of at least seven days' elevation and sometimes even more. In spite of the "torture" of being in the supine position for a week, I knew that the patient would be happier with his end result.

There are also other, more complicated ankle injuries. When an eversion injury rotates the fibula too far, its end (the lateral malleolus) can break (fracture). In theory, this is actually a better situation than one in which ligaments continue to rupture in an upward direction. In this case, only the tibio-fibular ligaments will be torn, and the fracture is minimally, if at all, displaced at the joint level. The fracture will heal, the ligament will heal, and because there is no instability with this injury, full recovery can be expected.

In some cases, however, the injuries are severe enough to fracture the fibula at its very top, near the knee joint. How does this happen? When all the ligaments from the ankle through the interosseous membrane to the upper leg have stretched and ruptured, the powerful forces can finally crack the fibula at its top. In any ankle injury with swelling and pain on both sides, the physician must examine not only the ankle but the entire fibula. If there is exquisite pain or crepitus about the fibula, an X-ray of the entire leg should be taken.

Most folks believe an ankle sprain is a simple problem needing minimal care. After which, they can go about their business as usual. This can certainly be the case, but in my experience, the situation is often not so simple. When all is said and done, many supposedly simple ankle sprains continue to cause pain, discomfort, and much frustration for both patient and doctor. If the doctor takes enough time to educate and communicate with the patient regarding the injury and its treatment, frustrations will be less, and the injured person will be more apt to cooperate, if he or she understands why aggressive but conservative treatment is the best approach.

It must be said, however, that even though the doctor may prescribe the proper treatment, and the patient complies fully with it, some lateral ligaments just don't heal well and remain looser than they were before the injury, a condition called *chronic lateral ankle instability*. The original injury need not even be severe for this to happen. With such an outcome, the person will continue to have repeated episodes of "turning my ankle" with the ankle giving way at the most inconvenient times. Repeat episodes are usually never as acute as the original injury, and the person may often carry on with whatever he was doing soon after the episode occurs. Taping and the use of a brace to control the inversion and eversion of the foot may suffice as treatment, but if the episodes begin to occur with daily activities and not just in sports, surgery to tighten these ligaments may be necessary.

Probably my most successful elective (non-emergency) operation was the one I did many times for a chronically unstable ankle: a modification of the Watson-Jones procedure using a small piece of the *peroneus brevis tendon* to reconstruct the original ligament by passing the tendon through bony tunnels tracing the injured ligaments responsible for lateral stability. All the patients were extremely happy with their results, and I can't recall anyone having more of the same trouble after the procedure. Other procedures now being used are just as successful, validating the medical adage, "Stick with what works best for you."

This is a subject on which I would like to expound a bit more. Many surgeons—and I include myself—are or have been swayed by new technological innovations that seem to appear monthly, especially in the field of orthopaedic surgery. It seems that some new instrument, device, or technique is always cropping up that looks promising, and anecdotal evidence of its success is mentioned. Human nature inclines the surgeon to grab on to one of these, and I was no exception when I was young. If it made sense, I bought it and used it on my next case. Sadly, I later learned that many of these innovations although they looked golden, soon lost their glitter and were no longer useful. Many a penny is being wasted on such novelties. A better approach would be to check out the innovation and, if it makes sense, watch for studies to prove its success and *then* buy it. Devices come and go, and they often become obsolete within a year. In other words, I let the other folks' successes and failures be my guide.

The same caution goes for new procedures as well. Surgeons who invent a way to treat a condition using new instrumentation often have ulterior motives, and the excellent results they present may not be matched by physicians following in their footsteps. All physicians need to be wary of falling into such situations. It's best to let others do the tinkering.

I remember a procedure someone developed for knees with a deficient anterior cruciate ligament (ACL). It was presented as an alternative to open ACL surgery, in the days before the arthroscopic technique was available. I performed the new procedure. It seemed to work well initially until, years later, some of those patients returned with another disability of the knee that was more difficult to treat than the original. This taught me a valuable lesson: wait until it's been proved that a procedure has good to excellent results before using it. I think it was Alexander Pope who counseled, "Be not the first by whom the new is tried, nor yet the last to lay the old aside." Pretty sound advice.

By now you may be thinking, *Well, he did try new surgical procedures to see if they would be successful, like the ones on the shoulder and the elbow.* Why, then, didn't I follow my own advice? First of all, no one had ever performed these specific surgeries. Also, I and others had done similar operations in the past, and I only modified the new methods using proven instrumentation. Finally, I always had the option of performing the older procedure in the event that I believed the newer technique would not succeed.

Lateral Synovial Impingement of the Ankle

This tongue-twisting name is one I came up with for a condition I encountered in a number of patients over the years. They always complained of pain in the front of the ankle toward the outside; some had no history of injury, while most had had a previous ankle sprain. Their physical findings were unremarkable except for the fact that I sometimes noted a thickening in the same area where they said they had pain. If I pressed that spot and manipulated the ankle, I could often reproduce their pain although I couldn't determine from that whether the problem was outside or inside the ankle.

After I injected lidocaine into the ankle, however, the pain almost immediately disappeared. Before the medication's effects wore off, I performed another careful examination of the ankle, and if the patient was still pain-free, I knew their pain was from inside the joint. If conservative treatment thereafter failed, I knew that an arthroscopic examination would reveal some disorder in the joint. Before undertaking the procedure, I told every patient what I expected to find, and that if I found anything else in the joint that could be causing the problem, I would deal with it at that time.

Once I had the patient's consent to proceed, what I found in all these cases was a fat pad on the outer side of the ankle joint, covered by a thickened scarred tissue that was also present between the talus and the tibia or between the talus and the fibula. Using low-intensity heat instrumentation, I was able to dissolve the fat pad and the synovium (the joint lining) while minimizing damage to surrounding healthy tissue, a simple operation to perform. Afterward, the patient was immediately able and actively encouraged to begin moving the ankle again. Most were quite satisfied with the results.

Osteochondritis Dissecans (OCD) of the Ankle

OCD of the talus is similar to OCD of the medial femoral condyle, which we discussed earlier. In the ankle, it is usually a result of trauma rather than a loss of blood supply. An ankle sprain can bruise the cartilage covering the talus, and continued motion inside the saddle joint will soften and possibly crack the cartilage, causing a cyst to form in the talus bone. Also, OCD can occur spontaneously with no previous injury. In either case, the blood supply is poor, and healing will be improbable. As in other joints—the knee, for example—this area of cartilage can also become detached from the surrounding bone, creating a defect on either the side or even the middle of the top of the talus (Fig. 67).

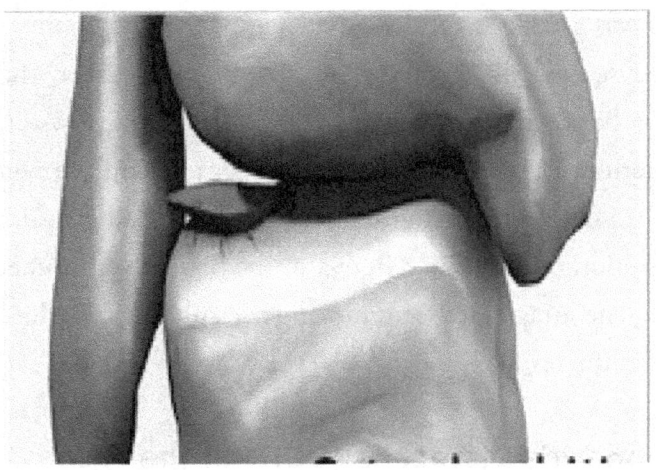

Fig. 67: OCD of the ankle involving the lateral aspect (left)
of the talus, loose but still intact
Image Courtesy of the Medical Multimedia Group LLC, www.eorthopod.com

Symptoms suggesting OCD include a dull or occasional sharp anterior pain in the ankle and the presence of more fluid than normal in the joint. If the person sits passively while the doctor manipulates the ankle, there may be no pain, and if only the hyaline cartilage—the cartilage at the bone ends forming joints—is involved, X-rays may not show a defect. Only after changes to the bone occur will X-ray examination reveal something amiss. After conservative treatment, if the pain persists and the physician has reason to suspect OCD, an arthroscopy of the ankle may be in order.

Subluxation or Dislocation of the Peroneal Tendon

Here's another condition I'm familiar with from having had it myself. I was fly-fishing on the Shenandoah River in Virginia, and as I stepped down with my foot firmly set against a rock, my ankle gave way, but without much pain. After I recovered my balance, it happened again and again. The discomfort was not terrible, but I seemed to have no control over my ankle, which is not the usual case with an ankle sprain. My wife came to

The Ankle

my rescue and helped me to shore, something she still reminds me of from time to time.

After removing my waders, I could see a significant difference between my left and right ankles. There was a bulge over my left lateral malleolus—the prominent roundish bone on the outside of the ankle—but none on my right. When I pressed gently on the bulge, it disappeared behind the bone, and I was able to walk and move my ankle. The improvement was short-lived, however, and the bulge soon came back, leaving my ankle seemingly unstable.

Knowing the anatomy of the joint, I recognized the bulging as my *peroneus* [pair-oh-NEE-us] *brevis tendon*, the extension of the *peroneus brevis muscle* that runs from the lower fibula to the base of the fifth metatarsal bone on the outside of the foot and plays a role in everting the foot, moving the foot outward. That tendon had ruptured its *peroneal retinaculum* [PAIR-oh-knee-al RET-tin-ack-cue-lum], an overlying fibrous band, allowing it to escape from its tunnel behind the lateral malleolus. It was then free to move forward, out, and over the malleolus until my pressing on it flipped it back into its groove.

Diagnosis made, I packed everything, drove home, and notified my partner that he had an emergency procedure to do that night. It's true that I could have sought medical attention where I was, to have the tendon pressed back into its groove and held there by a cast on my entire leg with the hope that it healed. I knew, however, that I wouldn't be able to tolerate a full leg cast for six weeks, and more important, I knew that casting wouldn't yield as good a result as an operation to reconstruct the top of the tunnel. At surgery that night, my partner replaced the tendon in its correct position and then repaired the torn ligamentous structure holding the tendon in place and put me in a cast for three weeks, followed by another three weeks in a removable boot. The rehabilitation period was quite short, and I didn't miss much time from the office and the operating room. To my relief, the surgery was a resounding success. That injury happened twenty years ago, and I've had no trouble from it since.

I mention this injury and have gone to great lengths to describe it because it often masquerades as a sprained ankle. Subsequent treatment for a sprained ankle will not produce a satisfactory outcome and could make a surgical reconstruction more difficult and cause a prolonged rehabilitation.

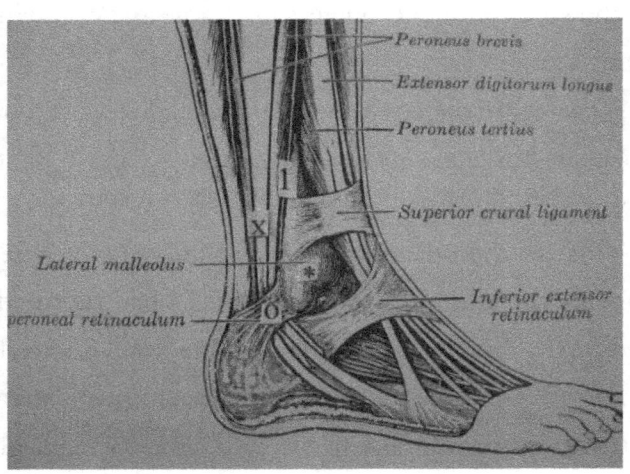

Fig. 68: Peroneal tendons behind the lateral malleolus (distal fibula) (*).
Peroneus longus tendon (x); peroneus brevis tendon (1).
Note fascial covering, retinaculum (o).
Gray's Anatomy, 1966

Posterior Tibialis Tendinits

By now, when you see a word ending in *-itis*, you know we're talking about inflammation, and when the word begins with *tendin-*, you know we're talking about a tendon. The *tibialis* [tib-ee-AL-lis] *posterior tendon* runs from the back of the calf down behind the medial malleolus, the short bony extension of the tibia forming the inside wall of the ankle saddle described earlier. This tendon passes into the middle inside part of the foot to attach to one of the tarsal bones, the *navicular* [nah-VICK-cue-lar].

One of its functions is to help support the arch of the foot, while its other main function is to invert the foot, turning the foot inward and up to a small degree. Its function is opposite that of the peroneus brevis (Fig. 68), which everts the foot, turning it outward and up a bit. In fact, for just about every muscle in the body, some other muscle serves the opposite function. This provision for opposition is more evidence of the marvelous design of the human body, as it is absolutely necessary to balance the joints to maintain function and stability. An excessive pull by one muscle, unless opposed equally by another, will certainly disturb the balance of the joint and cause some disorder.

The tibialis posterior tendon is yet another tendon that can suffer inflammation in the absence of any direct known cause. As with other tendons we've discussed, the inflammation can weaken the tendon, fragment its inner core, and cause an overall stretching that impairs the tendon's ability to function, with the result that the arch of the foot will gradually drop, making for a flatter foot.

Its first symptoms may be pain on the inner side of the ankle just behind or under the medial malleolus that continues to the side of the foot's arch. Some thickening may also be apparent in the area of the tendon, occasionally with redness. As the tendon stretches, the ankle will tend to roll inward, as with the pronated foot in Fig. 64, and the foot will become flatter as the normal curvature of the arch disappears. Arthritis may then develop in the foot and, in more severe cases, in the ankle itself.

Because the process is progressive, as soon as these symptoms appear, the person should be evaluated by an orthopaedist and followed closely thereafter. In many cases, treatment can begin with non-surgical approaches that may include any of the following: orthotic devices (supportive insoles for the shoes), bracing to give the arch more support (for example, an ankle stirrup brace), immobilization with a short-leg cast or boot to keep the person from bearing weight on that foot until healing occurs, physical therapy, non-steroidal anti-inflammatory drugs (NSAIDs), and custom-made shoes. If injections of refined steroid are used, they must go into the tendon sheath close to the diseased area, not into the tendon itself, and the fluid should be allowed to drift down around the tendon with the help of gravity.

In certain cases, however, surgery may be required. Surgical treatment may include just a *debridement*, trimming, and removing the degenerative tissue of the tendon, actual repair of the tendon, or realignment of the bones of the foot to recreate an arch. Results from these operations will certainly vary depending on the severity of the condition.

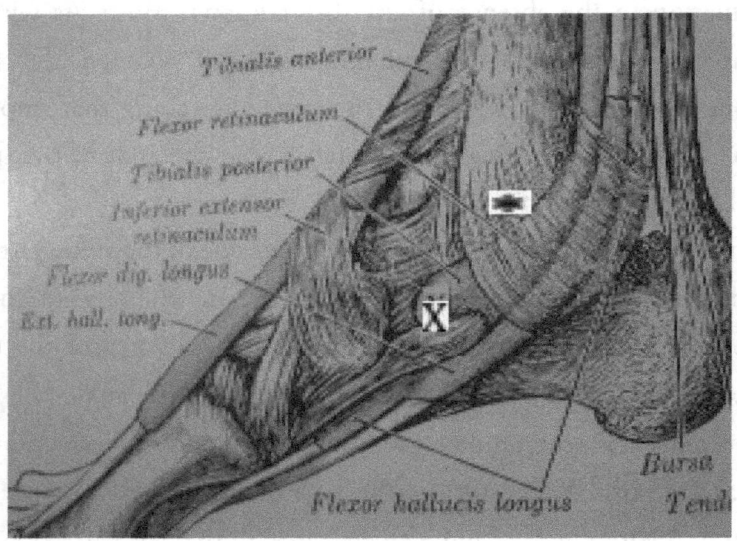

Fig. 69: Medial Side (inside) of Ankle: The tibialis posterior tendon is marked x. Medial malleolus (*).
Gray's Anatomy, 1966

Tarsal Tunnel Syndrome

We've already discussed the carpal-tunnel syndrome of the hand. The foot has a corresponding condition known as *tarsal tunnel syndrome*. It is much less common than the condition in the hand, and for that reason, you may have never heard of it. Its symptoms can be confused with those of tibialis posterior tendinitis as the involved nerve, the posterior tibial nerve, accompanies this same tendon through a tunnel behind the medial malleolus and is very closely related to the tendon in this area.

With this condition, compression or pinching of involved structures can produce pain and swelling similar to that occurring with the tendinitis. But in this case, because it's the nerve that's irritated and not the tendon, the person will complain of a burning pain, usually worse as the day progresses and usually relieved by rest, elevation, or massage. The patient may also report numbness and tingling sensations, and the doctor may be able to reproduce these by tapping over the nerve. This is known as a *Tinel's sign*. The posterior tibial nerve splits into two branches as it enters the foot, the medial and the lateral plantar nerves. Either branch or both can be affected. The doctor's sensory examination should reveal which branch is involved.

Rest, massage, applications of wet heat, physical therapy, and NSAID medications may help relieve the symptoms. Rarely, a surgical procedure to release the *laciniate* [lah-SIN-ee-ate] *ligament*, the covering over the tunnel that contains the nerve, will be necessary to relieve the compression on the nerve.

CHAPTER 17
THE FOOT

Plantar Fasciitis

The inner aspect of the heel bone is usually the area affected by *plantar fasciitis* [FAS-she-eye-tis] (Fig. 70). The word *plantar* refers to the sole of the foot, while *-itis* again means inflammation, therefore an inflammation of the fascia, the thick tendinous tissue that originates at the bottom of the heel bone and spreads toward the toes. Two layers of tissue cover the fascia at the heel: the skin and the fat pad under the heel. They play no part in this disorder.

We know of no specific cause for this inflammation although tension seems to be at the root of it. The plantar fascia extends like a bowstring along the length of the sole of the foot, and ill-fitting shoes, an inadequate arch, overuse, and being overweight have all been blamed for placing it under tension. If there is such tension, it will eventually pull on the fascia at the point where it connects to the heel bone, producing inflammation of both fascia and the bone's lining, periosteum. Over time, this traction irritates the periosteum enough to cause it to lay down bone in the direction of the traction to form a bone spur, or osteophyte. This bone spur is *NOT* the cause of the inflammation and traction. It is a result of it.

By the time all this has occurred, the person will be complaining of pain, stiffness, or severe aching in the area where the plantar fascia arises from the heel bone. The pain and stiffness are especially bad in the morning because the foot is relatively still overnight during sleep and as a result more inflammation and swelling build up. Thus those first steps in the morning bring immediate pain, lasting until the foot has been used enough to let the fascia stretch out. The pain may then disappear or, at least, become more bearable. It can affect both feet, although usually only one foot is affected at a time.

Treatment for plantar fasciitis includes almost everything under the sun: stretching exercises, heat, ultrasound, electrical stimulation, cortisone injections, devices to support the arch and heel, night splints to keep the fascia stretched, shock-wave therapy, laser treatments, and surgery. The long and short of it is, however, that none of these methods really cures the disorder, and experience has shown me that it must simply run its course. Newer techniques have illustrated long term good results, but I have no experience with them. Some folks do respond well to one or another of these treatments in less than two years, but as a general rule, the process will resolve itself, and the pain will disappear after twenty-four months. This disorder has affected both my own heels, and as a patient, I have undergone all the treatments mentioned except shock-wave therapy, laser treatments, and open surgery. In two years, the misery vanished, much to my relief.

Only a small number of people are willing to undergo an operation known as *plantar fasciotomy* in which the surgeon detaches the plantar fascia from the heel bone. This procedure is a last resort when the pain is severe and all else has failed, and a potential complication of the operation is that it may weaken the arch of the foot. I have heard of some good results from shock-wave therapy and laser surgery, but as I have said, I have no experience with them.

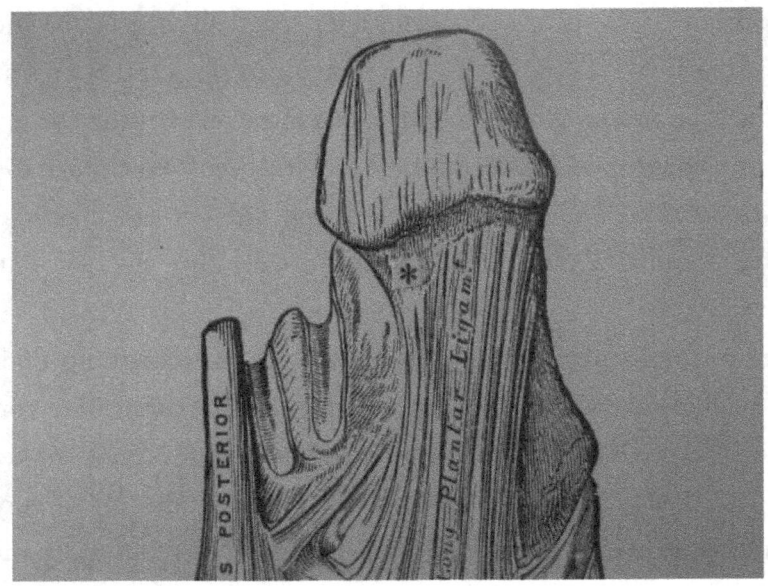

Fig. 70: Undersurface view (looking at the bottom) of plantar fascia origin on the right heel bone, calcaneus. * marks the area of the center of plantar fasciitis.

Pes Planus or Flat Foot

Many folks have *pes planus* (the term means "flat foot") but without symptoms. The normal arch of the foot is less evident or flatter, not having developed normally for some reason. Pes planus is not really a disease but rather a randomly occurring condition that can run in families. It can affect one or both feet and is most easily seen when the person stands with the entire sole of the foot in contact with the floor.

Two types exist, the rigid and the flexible. The flexible flat foot is easier to treat, if symptomatic, as the person can be fitted with orthotics that raise the arch. A rigid pes planus, on the other hand, cannot be helped by orthotics. Earlier, I referred to the acquired flat foot associated with problems of the tibialis posterior tendon. This is a flexible flat foot. With a rigid flat foot, bone deformation has occurred, not allowing any flexibility.

A third condition, not a true pes planus, may be seen in children whose concerned parents bring them to the pediatrician or orthopaedist, believing they have flat feet. The longitudinal arch of the foot does not fully form until the age of five in any child, and a fat pad under the skin and the arch in most of these children may mimic a true flat foot. Reassurance that the child does not have pes planus is all that is necessary. The parents should be told, however, that a pes planus may occur later in life but will have no relationship to this childhood appearance, or will any treatment at this early age have any effect.

Toeing-In Conditions

Metatarsus Adductus

Metatarsus adductus [Met-ta-tar-sus Ad-duct-tus] is a common foot deformity, usually noted at birth, that causes the front part of the foot (the forefoot) to turn inward. It, too, can be rigid or flexible. There is no known cause. Boys and girls are affected equally.

It is entirely possible that this condition will disappear on its own. Treatments include following the infant's condition, passive stretching exercises performed by the parents, corrective reverse-last shoes connected by a bar (Denis-Browne splint) for infants not yet walking, casting followed by straight-last shoes (shoes with no inward curve), and surgery. Surgery is usually reserved for the rigid or stiff metatarsus adductus, a rare condition.

Internal Tibial Torsion

All children are born with some internal tibial torsion, meaning that the tibia is spirally twisted slightly inward to some degree along its length, causing the feet to turn in or look "pigeon-toed." As the child grows, the twisting tends to unwind and the toeing-in disappears. In most children, this process is well on its way to unwinding within twelve months after they first walk, but the final resolution of the process may take years, with some residual toeing-in that requires no treatment.

We used to use a Denis-Browne splint for such conditions in infants until studies proved that doing nothing was just as useful. My biggest challenge in treating these kids was trying to convince the parents that no treatment was necessary. I never saw a case in which surgery was indicated.

Femoral Anteversion

In an adult, the head and neck of the femur are set off from the rest of the femur at an angle of about 15 degrees (Fig. 71). We call this the degree of *femoral anteversion*, angled forward or anteriorly.

All children are born with a much greater angle, somewhere from 45–60 degrees. When the angle is this high and the leg and the foot point straight ahead, the femoral head fits poorly into its pelvic socket. To fit better, the femur rotates inward, and the leg and the foot turn inward, creating a toeing-in appearance.

As the child grows and the angle gradually decreases to the normal 15 degrees, the toeing-in normally disappears. Let's say, on average, there's a normal correction over time of 30 degrees, so those children at 45 degrees will show no toeing-in when fully grown, but those who started at 60 degrees will have some residual toeing-in because they still have some "unnatural" anteversion present. This is not a bad thing. It will not lead to arthritis or gait problems. Most children get along fine even though they may still toe in to some degree when tired. Again, it's difficult to convince the parents that the condition will correct itself, and that their child may still exhibit some toeing-in in the future but will not require treatment.

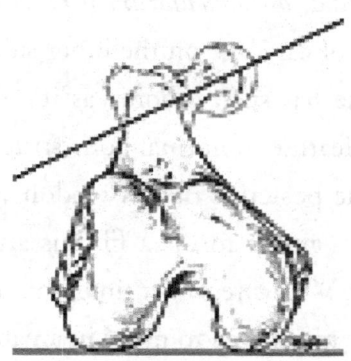

Fig. 71 Femoral anteversion: viewing the femur from the knee end to the hip end above. Note the 15 degree angle at which the femoral head and neck meet the adult femur
www.hopkinsortho.com/femoral_anteversion

Sinus Tarsi Syndrome

The *sinus tarsi* is an oblong tunnel or concavity of sorts between the talus and the calcaneus on the outside side of the foot (Fig. 66), over the subtalar joint. This tunnel contains ligaments that tie the talus and the calcaneus together, along with some fat, synovium, and a small nerve that runs to the skin on the outside of the foot just in front of the lateral malleolus, the outside ankle bone. If you feel that area of your own foot, it should be easy to identify.

Minor injuries, chronic ankle sprains, gout, and rheumatoid arthritis can cause this area to become painful. Diagnosing sinus tarsi syndrome is relatively simple because pressure directly over the sinus tarsi entrance will elicit the patient's complaint. The usual methods of treatment apply to this condition as well, and an injection of lidocaine and refined steroid will often relieve the symptoms. Surgery is almost never an option.

Accessory Navicular Bone

An accessory navicular, *os navicularum* [Os na-vick-you-LAIR-um], is an extra bone or piece of cartilage on the inner side of the foot just above the arch. Not everyone has such a bone, as it's a developmental oddity present at birth, not a feature of normal bone structure. The extra piece of bone is enclosed by the posterior tibialis tendon where it attaches to the normal navicular bone, and it forms a fibrous attachment or false joint with the true navicular. With stress over time, this attachment may loosen, and the accessory bone may begin to move in an abnormal fashion against the navicular bone, causing pain and possibly irritation of the posterior tibialis tendon irritation above it.

The examining physician will find an obvious bony prominence on the inner side of the foot, just above the arch, and any attempt to grasp it and move it may reproduce the patient's pain. Sometimes, there will also be redness and swelling. X-rays may reveal the extra bone, but if it is cartilage rather than bone, the X-ray will be normal.

Again, the usual conservative orthopaedic treatments are appropriate, but if the symptoms continue to bother the patient, surgery may be appropriate. Removing the accessory bone may be all that's required, although a repair of the posterior tibial tendon to improve its function may also be necessary. Removal of this extra bone does not usually affect the function of the foot thereafter.

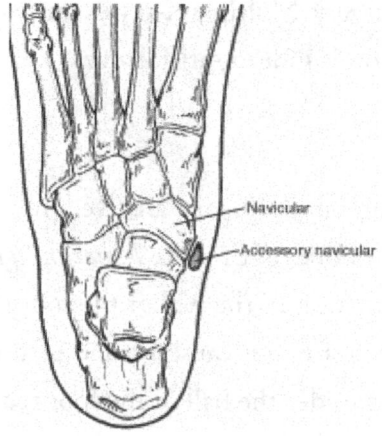

Fig. 72: Accessory navicular on medial side of the foot
next to the navicular bone
Courtesy of the American College of Foot and Ankle Surgeons

Lisfranc Subluxation, or Dislocation of the Foot

The assemblage of connected tarsal bones with the five metatarsals in the foot, which constitutes the main articulation of the forefoot and the mid-foot, carries the name the *Lisfranc joint* to honor a French surgeon of the eighteenth century. Lisfranc joint injuries include dislocations, subluxations, and fracture. They are often undiagnosed or misdiagnosed, causing later disabilities, including arthritis and, worst of all, chronic, unrelenting foot pain.

For that reason, the physician should be highly suspicious of any injury involving the top of the foot. Injuries to this area can be a mild sprain or a total dislocation without fracture. Abnormal swelling seen with a normal X-ray, any abnormal motion of the mid-foot on physical examination, pain and tenderness along any part of the Lisfranc joint, and black and blue areas on the sole of the foot—indicating blood under the arch—are all signs of a possible Lisfranc joint injury.

If a Lisfranc joint injury seems likely, the foot should be stabilized immediately, by either a closed reduction (bones manipulated into place without surgery) or surgery. Multiple X-ray examinations will be needed to make sure the reduction is indeed satisfactory.

Metatarsalgia

The metatarsals [me-tah-TAR-sals] are five long tubular bones between mid-foot bones and the bones of the toes. *Metatarsalgia* [Me-tah-tar-sal-jah] means pain and dysfunction of the ball of the foot (Fig. 73) (-*algia* means "pain"). Metatarsalgia has many causes, none of them primary. I believe that part of the fat pad under the ball of the foot reduces in thickness with age, and in conjunction with excessive physical activity, the wearing of ill-fitting shoes or mal-alignment of the foot, a loss of the fatty tissue cushion can create undue pressure over the ball of the foot (*metatarsal heads*) with irritation of the bursa in this area, causing bursitis (Fig. 73). The affliction happens more often in those with pes cavus, high-arched feet, and those with long second or short first metatarsal bones.

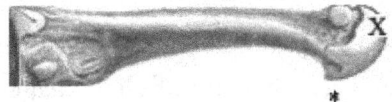

Fig. 73: A metatarsal bone. x marks the metatarsal head and
* marks the area of the bursitis of metatarsalgia.
Gray's Anatomy, 1966

Initially, it may feel as if something has lodged between the foot and the shoe, and the pain eventually worsens, usually under the end of the second metatarsal bone where it joins the second toe. The third and fourth metatarsal heads may be involved as well. Weight-bearing causes pain, and standing or walking in bare feet may have the same effect. The first symptoms and aching in the entire foot, especially the ball, often develop while standing for a great length of time.

Treatment can vary, from rest and application of ice for an acute onset to heat, massage, and staying off one's feet for a while for chronic foot pain. If the pain continues, NSAIDs, shock-absorbing insoles, proper shoes with good arch support to keep the foot from pronating, and metatarsal pads placed behind the metatarsal heads to relieve the pressure may help.

Rarely, an osteotomy—an operation to cut the metatarsal bone and raise the head out of its plantar-flexed position—may be necessary. Some physicians use a so-called floating osteotomy with no fixation, allowing the metatarsal to heal at its own height as the patient bears weight. Others advocate using rigid fixation to control the position of the metatarsal head.

Morton's Neuroma

Here's another of those disorders named for the physician who first described it. A *Morton's neuroma*, oddly enough, is not a true neuroma. The word *neuroma* means "a tumor of a nerve." A more correct name for the condition is *perineural fibrosis* [PERRY-neur-ral FY-bro-sis] to describe chronic scar tissue (*fibrosis*) surrounding (*peri-*) a nerve (*neural*, meaning "relating to a nerve"). It almost always occurs between the third and fourth metatarsal heads, probably from compression of the digital nerve serving the outer side of the third toe and the inner side of the fourth toe. (The word *digital* refers to the digits—fingers and toes.) I have never seen one between the first and second toes, or the fourth and fifth.

Why does it happen only in the third web space? This particular nerve differs from the foot's other digital nerves in that it comprises branches from two other nerves, so it may therefore be slightly larger than the other digital nerves. Its size and position make it more vulnerable to irritation from rubbing against the deep ligaments that hold the base of the toe joints together. Even so, I don't believe the metatarsal heads truly compress this nerve. Rather, I think the irritation builds up, forming more scar tissue and causing even more irritation—a vicious circle.

Symptoms include pain in the third and forth toes and numbness and tingling in the areas of skin this nerve supplies. Conservative treatment may include wider shoes and a metatarsal pad just behind the third and fourth metatarsal heads to help spread them apart during weight-bearing. Local cortisone injections may reduce the inflammation and thickening of the nerve enough to eliminate the pain. Treatment may also include a metatarsal bar for the shoe, shifting pressure from the painful joints or a rocker-bottom sole. Some physicians believe a rigid shoe sole will relieve pressure on all the metatarsal heads. As one of my orthopaedic foot surgeon friends once said in regard to conservative treatment, "Don't do what hurts, until it doesn't hurt to do it anymore." His wisdom really sums up most of what there is to say about treating this condition conservatively.

But conservative treatment may not solve the problem, and surgery may be necessary because of the mechanics involved in the process. Two types of surgeries may be considered. The surgeon may either make an incision in the transverse metatarsal ligament, leaving the nerve alone or remove the digital nerve itself. Good results can be expected with either of these procedures in 80 percent of cases, but before agreeing to the operation, all patients must understand that there's a 20 percent chance of a poor result.

Hallux Valgus or Bunion

Hallux means "large toe," and *valgus* or *valgum* means "tilted outward away from the midline" of the body. If something is tilted inward from the body's midline, we use the term *varus or varum*. We refer to a knock-kneed person, for example, as having *genu* ("knee") *valgum*, and a bow-legged person we describe as having *genu varum*.

Hallux valgus (Fig.74) forms when the big toe tilts toward the second toe rather than pointing straight ahead. This tends to shift the first metatarsal head out of alignment, away from the second metatarsal bone, producing a classic bunion bump or protuberance. Bunions progress over time, tilting little by little, with gradual thickening and increased prominence of the tissues over the protuberance. If there are symptoms, they usually appear later. Tight or pointed shoes don't necessarily cause bunions, but they can certainly make the deformity worse and cause symptoms earlier. In my practice, because I saw many more women with bunions than men, I always thought their footwear had to be a major contributing factor.

Typical symptoms are inflammation, soreness, pain, redness, and thickening over the inside portion of the big toe joint. Treatments include shoes that have a wide toe box. All pointed toe or high-heeled shoes should be eliminated from the wardrobe. NSAID medications, custom-made shoes, and cutout pads over the bunions are also options. Injections are rarely used as they affect only the bursa and do nothing for the deformity. Some patients will respond to conservative treatment and, when they no longer have pain, return to wearing the shoes that added to their problem in the first place. This is one of the most frustrating problems I encountered while treating bunions. The pain and disability almost always recurred.

Several surgical procedures are done for bunions, all designed to correct the deformity by removing the protuberance and straightening the first metatarso-phalangeal joint, the joint at the base of the big toe. I won't go into the various procedures available. If you have a bunion, your physician will evaluate it and choose the best procedure for that specific deformity. Please remember that not all surgeries work, and surgeries on feet, if unsuccessful, can lead to a chronically painful result.

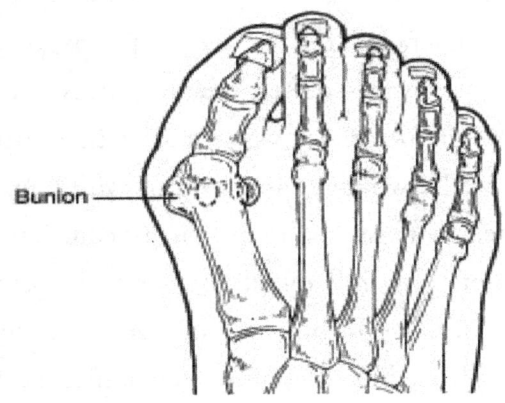

Fig. 74: Hallux valgus or bunion
Courtesy of the American College of Foot and Ankle Surgeons

Bunionette or Tailor's Bunion

A so-called *bunionette* [BUN-yun-et] or *tailor's bunion* is a deformity similar to a true bunion, occurring on the outer side of the fifth metatarsophalangeal joint at the base of the small toe (Fig.75), but it is not as common as a bunion of the big toe. Years ago, tailors often developed such deformities from sitting cross-legged on the floor for long periods of time with the outer side of the small toe pressed against the floor. Although tailors rarely sit this way today, the name for the disorder persists. A tailor's bunion can also be caused by a muscle imbalance or the wearing of ill-fitting shoes. Symptoms of tailor's bunion/bunionette include redness, swelling, and pain at the site of the enlargement, particularly when wearing shoes that rub the outside of the foot, irritating the soft tissues under the skin and producing inflammation.

A better-fitting shoe to accommodate the width of the foot is usually all that's needed to remedy the problem although the usual conservative treatments for inflammation can help. If doctor and patient agree that an operation is indicated, however, it will generally have excellent results.

The Foot

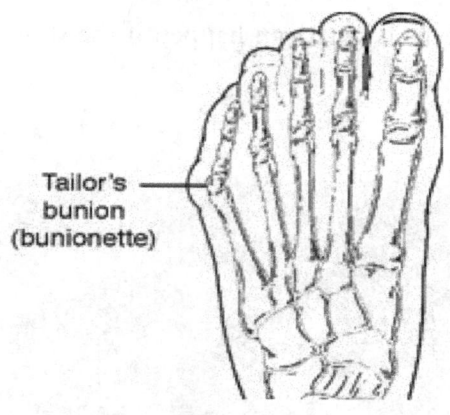

Fig. 75: Tailors bunion or bunionette.
Courtesy of the American College of Foot and Ankle Surgery

Hammertoes and Claw Toes

Hammertoe and claw-toe deformities are caused by an intrinsic imbalance of the toe muscles. They occur five times more often in women than in men. With at least six sets of muscles controlling each toe, it's no wonder that somewhere along the line, especially with age, some of these muscles may overpower others. Besides the muscles, each toe contains three bones or *phalanges* [FA-lan-geez] (singular, *phalanx*). The first bone extending from the metatarsal is called the proximal phalanx, next is the middle phalanx, and last is the distal phalanx.

So how does a hammertoe deformity occur? If the first muscle to contract is the short muscle responsible for flexing a toe, the *flexor digitorum* [dij-it-TORE-um] *brevis*, it may overpower the rest of that toe's muscles and pull the middle phalanx downward, bend the joint between the proximal and middle phalanges (*proximal inter-phalangeal* or PIP joint) upward, and cause the toe's last joint—the one between the middle and distal phalanges (*distal inter-phalangeal* or DIP joint)—to hyperextend or bend upward. The consequent distortion, known as a hammertoe (Fig. 76), can also cause bursitis under the metatarsal head, producing a metatarsalgia as we've already discussed. This is what can happen if the short flexor muscle acts first.

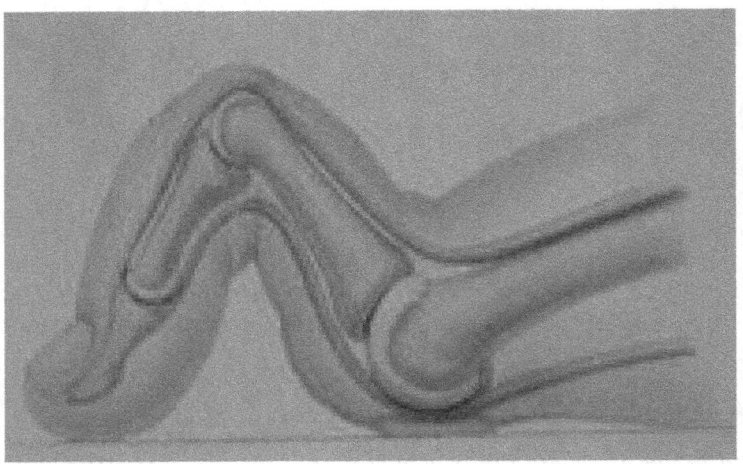

Fig. 76: Hammertoe. Note how bones stick up at the middle (PIP) joint

On the other hand, if the long flexor of the toe overpowers the smaller muscles, it can pull on the proximal phalanx, bending the outer two toe joints downward and back toward the sole to create the deformity known as claw toe. The difference between the two deformities is slight, caused by slightly different imbalances. In both conditions, painful calluses may form on top of the bones that stick up to rub against the shoe, perpetuating the pain cycle. Calluses may also form on the tip of the toes.

Treatment will include NSAID medications, padding, splinting, and manipulation to prevent rigid contractures, and custom orthotics and shoes to accommodate the deformity. Ultimately, surgery may be necessary to correct the deformity, either an arthroplasty to create a new PIP joint or an arthrodesis (fusing) of this joint.

Ingrown Toenail

An *ingrown toenail* is just what it says—a nail whose edge has grown into the surrounding soft tissue. While this might not seem like something an orthopaedist would deal with, many folks with other orthopaedic issues also have ingrown toenails, and because they can cause considerable discomfort, an orthopaedist or a podiatrist is often the first responder. Believe me, an ingrown nail is not something to be taken lightly, especially in someone with diabetes, poor circulation, or the start of an infection. Failure to treat it properly can have dire consequences.

Ingrown toenails happen most commonly after the nails are improperly cut. On occasion, the toenail may start to curve, bowing upward in its center so that its edges cut down into the skin as the nail grows. Cutting a toenail too short encourages the skin next to the nail to grow over the nail, eventually causing the normal crease between nail and soft tissue to disappear. Then as the nail grows out, it cuts into the skin, making a break that a bacteria can enter, causing pain, redness, and swelling. I have also seen a toe with ingrown nail on both sides.

The proper way to cut toenails is straight across, not rounded at the corners and not too short. It's best to leave them a little long rather than cutting too close. Large toenail clippers are the best tool to use, not smaller clippers designed for fingernails. And making several small cuts is preferable to trying to do it in one cut. In spite of proper cutting, some toenails just seem to want to grow into the flesh no matter what. Some folks find it helpful to wedge a tiny piece of absorbent cotton soaked in rubbing alcohol under the nail corners immediately after cutting, encouraging the nail to grow out straight.

Another cause of ingrown toenails is wearing shoes that are too tight or too short. An ingrown nail can also form after an injury that makes the nail grow in a cup shape rather than the normal slightly convex form.

Treatment is always directed first at an infection, if present. The first step is antibiotic medication given by mouth for ten days in the hope that the redness and swelling will disappear. In my practice, I always checked the patient again after two more weeks to be sure the infection had been eliminated. If the problem was likely to be ongoing, I suggested surgery. One approach is to trim back the offending nail as a preliminary attempt to correct the nail's curvature. If this fails, the next step is to remove part or all of the nail and destroy the nail bed from which it grows. Patients must be made aware, however, that there may be some residual growth of the nail if a small or even microscopic portion of the nail bed is left behind.

CHAPTER 18
STRESS FRACTURES

I said at the beginning that I wouldn't discuss fractures, but stress fractures are really a different breed. These fractures don't occur as a result of an immediate injury but come on gradually as stresses build up within the bone from running or some repetitive weight-bearing activity.

I equate it with bending a paper clip that's been straightened out. One bend and even several bending motions don't affect the integrity of the metal, but continued bending of the clip over time creates a stress within the metal to build until the metal finally breaks.

The same thing happens with bone. Bone will tolerate running one day or several days well, but over time, stress in some bones builds up in certain areas until the bone reacts like the paper clip. If you observe the clip as it nears its breaking point, you can see changes in the metal. The bone reacts the same way, and eventually a crack appears that weakens the bone. A through-and-through fracture may follow. For that reason, it's important to be suspicious of pain in anyone performing an intense training program or running long distances repetitively.

Stress fractures are a common problem, especially in runners and military recruits. These fractures may occur with as little as two or three weeks of training, can be very mild, and may cause only minimal changes to the bone, which eventually heals. On the other hand, they may progress to the point of a complete fracture that requires surgical repair.

Uncommon complications can occur as well. Two areas of great concern in this regard are the femoral neck (the portion of bone directly under the ball of the hip joint) and the front side of the tibia. Symptoms suggestive of a stress fracture must be given due consideration until some other diagnosis is found that accounts for the difficulties.

A stress fracture of the femoral neck is one of the most difficult fractures to diagnose. The pain may be poorly localized in the groin, or it may be referred to the thigh or the knee as I pointed out in an earlier chapter. Physical findings are minimal at best, and diagnostic X-rays may reveal nothing at all. The next level of investigation should be a bone scan, followed by an MRI, if the bone scan reveals nothing.

Failure to diagnose such a fracture may have terrible consequences, including *avascular necrosis*, a loss of blood supply with death and deterioration of the femoral head. Because blood is supplied to the femoral head by way of the femoral neck, a fracture of the femoral neck may disrupt the blood supply to the femoral head. Bone death and collapse of the femoral head may follow, necessitating a total hip replacement. Hip replacements are usually reserved for older patients, but what's so terrible about this condition is that the folks who develop it usually are young and very athletic. One should be highly suspicious of a femoral neck stress fracture when the suggestive symptoms appear in an athletic young person.

About 5–10 percent of stress fractures are in the femoral neck. The first and more common type is a stress fracture on the *compression* side, the inferior (bottom) aspect. The second, less common type is a stress fracture on the *tension* side, the superior (top) aspect. As the top of the femoral neck is convex, or curved upward, repetitive activity can create a force that pushes down or stretches, placing tension along the convex (cup-shaped) curvature. Continued tension will eventually cause a crack, hence a *tension stress fracture*. On the other hand, those same forces, if measured, would tend to compress the line on the bottom concave curvature of the femoral neck, and the compression will cause a crack in the bone here, hence a *compression stress fracture*.

Tension stress fractures in the hip are best-treated with surgery to pin and stabilize the femoral neck so the tension forces don't completely break through the bone. Compression stress fractures can be treated by immediate avoidance of weight-bearing for eight to fourteen weeks. At that point, X-rays should show bone healing with new white bone on the inferior neck. A bone scan, which may still be hot in this area, is not a good measure of the progression of healing.

Should a through-and-through fracture occur (a *displaced femoral-neck fracture*), immediate surgery is necessary to decompress the blood inside the joint and stabilize the fracture as anatomical as possible. Unfortunately, avascular necrosis may occur with or without early surgery, but operating immediately may help reduce the likelihood of necrosis.

Other stress fractures can also happen in the neighborhood of the hip. One vulnerable area is the *pubic rami* [RAY-my] *of the pelvis*. Pain arising from these structures forming part of the front of the pelvis is rather like pain originating in the femoral neck. Here's another reason why it's so important for the doctor to rule out a stress fracture of the femoral neck. Fractures of the pubic rami are usually not displaced and will heal on their own with rest and a period of minimal weight-bearing.

Stress fractures have also been identified in the greater trochanter, that knobby part of the top of the femur we described before. These are usually not displaced either, but they do cause pain similar to that originating in the femoral neck and that arising from a greater trochanteric bursitis. A bone scan will help to differentiate this fracture from a fracture of the pelvis or the hip.

Another site for a possible stress fracture is the femur, usually on its front side midway along its shaft. If misdiagnosed, such a stress fracture could cause serious difficulties. A complete fracture through the femur will become displaced, requiring immediate surgery. If the femoral stress fracture can be diagnosed before the bone fractures through and through, the surgeon can perform an elective operation to stabilize the bone known as *intramedullary nailing*, placing a metallic device down the middle of the bone. This operation is much easier than the procedure required for a through-and-through displaced fracture and promotes earlier healing.

The symptom of a tibial stress fracture (Fig. 77) is pain around the front midshaft of the shinbone. As with other types of stress fracture, bony changes may or may not appear on X-ray. Treatment may include an air splint, which is a plastic support with a soft inflatable inner bladder, a patellar-tendon bearing cast or casting the entire leg to immobilize the tibia above and below the fracture until the patient is pain-free and shows evidence of good healing on X-ray. Most of these treatments succeed, but in cases with persistent pain after six months, intramedullary nailing of the tibia with possible grafting may be needed. This particular area is known to have a poor blood supply so in the event that a tibial stress fracture fails to heal (nonunion), nailing and bone grafting is definitely the preferred treatment. In some cases of nonunion, success with electrical bone stimulation has been documented, but most orthopaedists would opt for the surgical intervention.

Stress Fractures

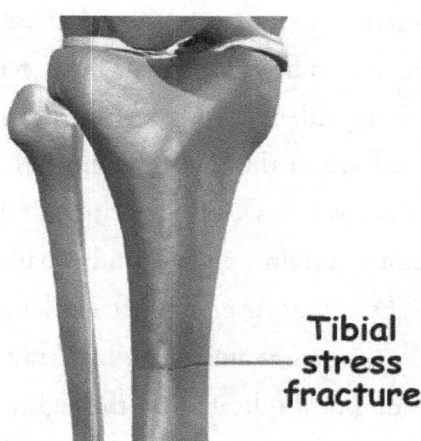

Fig. 77: Tibial stress fracture.
Image courtesy of Medical Multimedia Group LLC,
www.eOrthopod.com

Another bone that can suffer a stress fracture is the fibula, the smaller long bone of the lower leg. Runners can have such fractures, which usually heal in four to six weeks with conservative therapy, rarely requiring surgery.

Stress fractures occur also in the navicular bone of the foot, located just below the ankle joint as described in the previous chapter. Running can transmit repetitive forces to the foot directly through this bone. Pain from a stress fracture of the navicular bone is almost always directly over the bone, which can be quite tender and painful on examination. Six weeks in a short-leg non-weight-bearing cast, followed by four to six weeks in a weight-bearing cast, is usually all that's needed to heal the condition. Afterward, a gradual return to full weight-bearing with a semirigid shoe is usually allowed.

Finally, what is probably the most common of all stress fractures can occur in the metatarsal bones of the foot. The second metatarsal is most frequently involved, but all the metatarsals can be affected. The examining doctor can easily identify tenderness over the fracture, most commonly at the mid-shaft. Wearing a cast for four to six weeks is usually all that's needed for these fractures to heal. Surgery is rarely required.

I have one interesting sidenote on stress fractures. While all the stress fractures I've discussed are in the lower extremities, I did see one in the collarbone. The patient was a weightlifter in training for the Olympics and could not get past a certain weight with his daily lifting program. He complained of a slight aching over his left clavicle while lifting but no pain when he wasn't training. Examination by X-ray revealed a very slight change on the left side not duplicated on the right, and a bone scan was "hot" over the mid-shaft of his clavicle. Unfortunately, his Olympics trials were to take place too soon to allow complete healing of the fracture, so he never qualified to compete. His fracture healed, however, without any side effects.

CHAPTER 19
OSTEOPOROSIS

The word *osteoporosis* [OST-e-o-pore-os-sis] means "porous bone." Although it's a mighty big subject to tackle in one chapter, I'll attempt to lay out some basics about this disease that affects millions of people. There is a minor condition that precedes true osteoporosis called *osteopenia*, meaning that a little less bone structure is present than normal but not enough to be categorized as osteoporosis.

Bones contain minerals, and over time, they can lose minerals in a process called demineralization. This process can be tested with dual-energy X-ray absorptiometry (DEXA), a form of X-ray examination that can detect amounts of bone loss as small as 2 percent per year. Certain measurements detected by this test determine whether someone has normal mineralization of bone, osteopenia, or osteoporosis.

From the moment of birth, the human skeleton loses old bone and forms new bone. In our first two decades of life, we form new bone faster than we lose bone. Our bodies, therefore, form dense bone until *peak bone mass* is reached—the greatest amount of bone we'll ever have. That occurs around the age of twenty. Afterward, a slow change begins, with slightly more bone being lost than new bone formed. This process is very slow, but it happens in all of us, more quickly and more markedly in some people than in others. A growing imbalance of old bone lost and new bone formed occurs four or five times more often in women than in men, especially after menopause, when estrogen levels drop precipitously. Studies have shown that within four to five years after menopause, some women may lose up to 20 percent of their bony mass. Post-menopausal women given estrogen replacement therapy, on the other hand, may not have the same rate of bone loss as women who don't take the hormone.

To recap, osteoporosis occurs when too much bone is lost or too little is formed. Actually, both can happen at the same time. The more bone we have at the time of our peak bone mass, the better off we'll be once the rate of bone loss starts to overtake the rate of new bone formation.

If you were to look at normal bone tissue through a microscope, you would observe a thickness of the solid outer part (the *cortical* bone) while the inner bone (the *medullary* bone) would remind you of a honeycomb, with small vacant spaces. In osteopenia and osteoporosis, the honeycomb effect becomes more noticeable, the empty spaces larger than in normal bone, and the cortical bone thins out (Fig. 78). This loss of minerals and calcium weakens the bone and may lead eventually to fractured long bones and collapsed spinal vertebrae.

In osteoporosis, the loss of minerals and calcium is so much greater that, in some cases, the medullary bone retains very little bony latticework, and the cortical bone is obviously thinner than normal. This can be seen on a plain X-ray film.

Osteoporosis

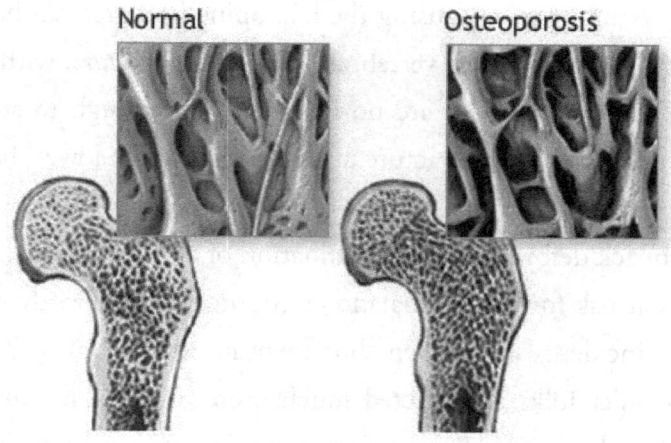

Fig. 78: Left: normal honeycomb appearance of normal bone. Right: osteoporosis with loss of bone and mineralization with thinning and weakening of bony structures.
www.healthallrefer.com

How does bone form? *Collagen* [KOLL-a-jin] is a framework on which bone is built. This protein-based material is initially loose and quite flexible. A combination of calcium phosphate and other minerals then reinforces the framework to form a rigid structure. Thereafter, a continuous reciprocal action occurs in which tiny bone-producing cells called *osteoblasts* [OSS-tee-oh-blasts] and bone-absorbing cells called *osteoclasts* [OSS-tee-oh-klasts] break down bone and rebuild it during every minute of our lives. Unfortunately, after the peak bone mass period, new bone builds up at a slower rate than the rate at which old bone is absorbed.

With osteopenia, one has no symptoms. Osteoporosis has few if any symptoms until a fracture occurs. Bones most commonly fractured from osteoporosis are the hip, the spine, and the wrist. The wrist is usually fractured in a fall. Hip fractures can also come about through a fall or through a sudden twisting of the lower extremity when the demineralized upper part of the femur gives way under the body's weight. Some physicians believe that in someone with known osteoporosis, the femur may fracture and give way on its own, causing the fall. Spine fractures can happen as a result of compression of the vertebrae, *compression fracture*, with no injury at all as if the spinal bones are no longer strong enough to support the weight of the body. Such a fracture usually occurs in the lower thoracic and upper lumbar vertebrae, causing loss of height, sometimes severe back pain or a hunchback deformity, or a combination of all these results.

Who is at risk for osteopenia and osteoporosis? I've already mentioned the higher incidence in women, but men are affected as well. It makes sense that older folks are affected much more often than younger ones, but not all older people have osteoporosis. It's important to know one's family history of the disease as heredity and genetics play a part in its onset and severity. Low estrogen levels in women and low testosterone and estrogen levels in men can be contributing factors. Smoking and alcohol consumption are risk factors. Diet is very important, especially with regard to the amounts of calcium, vitamin D, phosphorous, magnesium, vitamins B6 and B12, vitamin K, and protein consumed. Some foods and drinks—those with caffeine or too much salt, for example—can reduce calcium absorption. Some medications can also affect the absorption of calcium, especially oral and intravenous steroids, antacids that contain aluminum, cancer drugs, proton-pump inhibitors for acid reflux, and some birth control medications.

If you have a question about some of the medications you're taking, please ask your doctor. There are also diseases that cause osteoporosis, such as diabetes and malabsorption conditions of the gastrointestinal tract.

In general, anyone over fifty years of age should see his or her physician to learn how to prevent or minimize the effects of this disease. Osteoporosis can be prevented, but no cure is yet available. Seeing your physician is especially important if you have risk factors for it such as a positive family history or an unwise diet. Bone density testing can be done, always at the discretion of your physician, to help establish a baseline for comparison with future examinations. It also seems that vitamin D and calcium are absolutely necessary to help prevent and possibly reverse some osteoporosis. Neither one can do the job alone.

Some natural ways to help keep your bones strong are: get your Vitamin D level tested and try to keep a level of at least 120nmol, have a daily cup of beef/lamb bone broth, and add vitamin A rich cod liver oil to your supplements. If you can find it, drink one to two cups full cream raw milk. However, always discuss any of these with your physician before treating yourself.

Finally, a word about another disease *osteomalacia* [oss-tee-oh-mah-LAY-shee-ah], which means "soft bones." While osteoporosis is a demineralization and weakening of bone, osteomalacia comes about through a malfunction of the bone-building process. Much less prevalent than osteoporosis, osteomalacia is known in children as rickets. These children have bones that will bow and fracture because they have deficient vitamin D. One cause is insufficient exposure to the sun. Sun exposure helps the body produce the vitamin D needed to process and absorb calcium. Other causes are long term use of certain drugs such as anti-seizure medication, insufficient intake of vitamin D, certain intestinal operations that affect the absorption of calcium, and celiac disease, which affects the intestines and prevents absorption of vitamin D.

The symptoms of osteomalacia may be minimal to nonexistent, but as a general rule, signs of the disease not found with osteoporosis include muscle weakness in the arms and legs and bone aching in the lower spine, pelvis, and legs. Vitamin D supplements and other minerals will be needed to treat the disorder.

CHAPTER 20
FIBROMYALGIA

Fibromyalgia [FY-bro-my-al-ghea] means pain in fibrous and muscle tissue. The term *myofasciitis* [MY-o-fas-she-i-tis] also means the same thing. It's a chronic condition characterized by widespread pain in the muscles, ligaments, and tendons as well as general fatigue and multiple trigger points of pain where slight pressure on some part of the body can elicit pain. It occurs in 2 percent of the population in the United States. Women are affected more often than men, and the risk of developing fibromyalgia increases with age. Symptoms of fibromyalgia may come on after some physical or emotional trauma, but in most cases, the condition has no known cause.

Signs and symptoms of fibromyalgia vary, depending on the weather, stress, physical activity, and even time of day. Widespread pain and tender points are hallmarks of the condition. Someone who has the pain of fibromyalgia describes it as a constant dull ache, typically arising from muscles. For a true diagnosis of fibromyalgia, the affected person must have pain on both sides of the body and both above and below the waist. Trigger points typical of fibromyalgia include the following:

- Back of the head
- Between the shoulder blades
- Top of the shoulders

- Front sides of the neck
- Upper chest
- Outer elbows
- Upper hips
- Sides of the hips
- Inner knees

You may notice that all the trigger points listed are in areas I have mentioned in this book.

Fibromyalgia sufferers usually awaken tired. Researchers believe that such folks rarely reach the deep, relaxing stage of sleep. No one knows what causes fibromyalgia, but it most likely involves a variety of factors working together that may include at least the following:

- Genetics, as fibromyalgia tends to run in families
- Infection, as some illnesses appear to trigger or aggravate the condition
- Physical or emotional trauma, such as post-traumatic stress disorder

What is the mechanism of the pain? A theory of central sensitization maintains that the brains of people suffering from this condition have an abnormal reaction to pain and thus a lower threshold for it. An abnormal increase in levels of certain chemicals in the brain's transmitters suggests to researchers that repeated nerve stimulations alter the brains of fibromyalgia sufferers, leading the brain's pain receptors somehow to "remember" the pain more prominently and therefore become more sensitive and overreact to it.

Fibromyalgia is not progressive nor does it generally lead to other conditions or diseases. Effects of the disorder that impair one's ability to work or sustain personal relationships are depression and sleep deprivation. Patients often become increasingly frustrated with the vagueness of the diagnosis and subsequent attempts to treat their condition. The investigating doctor should check specific areas for tenderness, applying mild finger pressure just sufficient to whiten part of a nail bed. A specific diagnosis of fibromyalgia requires widespread pain lasting at least three months and at least eleven positive trigger points out of a possible eighteen. There is no lab test that can confirm this diagnosis, but studies of blood count, erythrocyte sedimentation rate (ESR), and thyroid function should be performed.

As for treatment of the disorder, such medications as acetaminophen, NSAIDs, antidepressants, and anti-seizure drugs have had beneficial effects. Pregabalin (Lyrica) is the first drug approved by the Food and Drug Administration for fibromyalgia treatment. Physical therapy to restore muscle balance may reduce pain. Stretching techniques, along with application of wet heat, ice, or both, may help. Cognitive behavioral therapy and counseling may help in dealing with stressful situations.

There's no question that many folks who have been told they have fibromyalgia actually have other disorders. Even though a patient may have many complaints, many of the specific symptoms mentioned in this book occur at same time and may mistakenly lead patients to think they have fibromyalgia. Some physicians, not so aware of the symptoms needed to make the final diagnosis of fibromyalgia, may mistakenly label the patient with this diagnosis. For instance, a patient can have tennis elbow, rotator-cuff problems, low back pain, a degenerative medial meniscus, and plantar fasciitis all at one time. That person definitely has many complaints and tender areas but doesn't have fibromyalgia.

Sometimes, a physician will try to lump a patient's numerous complaints into the one diagnosis of fibromyalgia. I call this a "wastebasket diagnosis." Such an attempt to cram everything under one label essentially robs the patient of specific treatment regimens for each of her diagnoses. Should this happen, the patient will then be labeled with a diagnosis of fibromyalgia for a very long time, and any treatments prescribed for the supposed fibromyalgia will not help the separate disorders. In other words, the physician must be very careful to examine the patient for individual medical conditions and rule them out before finally diagnosing fibromyalgia.

CHAPTER 21
BONE HEALING

A previous chapter touched on how and where common stress fractures occur. Of course, fractures of all sorts happen in most long bones of the body as well as some others. But how does a fracture heal? Answering this question could require another book, but I'll attempt to give you a quick tour of a fracture site to give you some idea how the process works.

Let's choose a fracture that is not displaced. What I mean by that is the two fragments are in a straight alignment and 100 percent contact, with no offset. If the periosteum, the layer covering the bone, is intact, most of the healing will be through cells in this tissue that lay down new bone when stimulated to do so. There will be some bleeding from the fracture site, forming a small hematoma. The blood in the hematoma will clot and form a fibrous mass that will be invaded initially by inflammatory cells, then by *fibroblast* [FY-bro-blast] *cells*, whose job is to produce *fibrin* [FY-brin], the tissue that forms an organized fibrous clot.

After that, an ingrowth of blood vessels and a migration of *mesenchymal* [mes-sen-KA-mall] cells that can differentiate into various types of cells invade the fibrin tissue. The primary oxygen supply of this early process comes from exposed *cancellous* [can-SELL-us], soft bone inside the rigid long bone and the periosteum. Because this reaction phase is primarily an inflammatory one, it's important to know that during this critical time, anti-inflammatory medications could work against the progress of healing.

Once the fibrous mending has taken place and the fibroblasts have laid down a bed of fibrin, or *stroma*, a repair phase begins. This stroma is a sort of meshwork or latticework that vascular cells and blood vessels infiltrate to bring oxygen and help nurture a living tissue that other cells will mineralize and calcify later. This fibrous formation forms a soft, pliant tissue—a *callus*—around the repair site. In the first four to six weeks of healing, this callus is quite weak and requires adequate protection in the form of a brace, a cast, and some device for external or internal fixation. Otherwise, the callus will become loose and pliable, not firmer. Eventually, it will become a rigid bony mass that forms a bridge of woven bone between the two fracture fragments.

Unless the fracture site is appropriately immobilized, the callus may not undergo mineralization and eventual ossification, and an unstable fibrous mass (nonunion) may develop instead. During the healing process, two other factors can also increase the risk of nonunion: taking anti-inflammatory medications for long periods and the lingering of nicotine in the body from smoking. Because nicotine constricts the blood vessels, it can inhibit the formation of the structures needed to supply nutrients and oxygen to the healing fracture. I always cautioned patients with healing fractures not to smoke, and I also gave the same advice to patients in need of successful bone healing for *whatever* reason.

Once fracture healing is complete, the remodeling phase begins with the healing bone attempting to restore the fracture site to its original shape and strength. This does not always result in a perfectly straight bone. Remodeling of the bone occurs over months or years, helped along by forces applied to the bone through axial mechanical stresses such as walking or bearing weight on the lower extremity. During this phase, bone is generally laid down where it is needed and resorbed or taken away from where it is not needed. Adequate strength is typically achieved in three to six months.

This remodeling phase occurs very quickly in children. It is so efficient, in fact, that the orthopaedist need not worry if a fracture exhibits some *angulation* when set, in other words, the break not quite in the normal straight alignment. For a child's healed fracture, the body will generally remodel and subsequently realign that angled repair until the bone appears to have never been broken. The younger the child, the more angle at the fracture one can accept. Of course, the doctor should attempt to set all fractures as anatomical as possible, but occasionally, it's impossible because the fracture is either oblique or comminuted (has more than two fragments). For this reason, few children's fractures need surgical repair although there are some that do, especially when they involve the growth centers of the elbow, hip, and knee.

Nonunions of fractures are uncommon although the tibia is quite prone to nonunion. Nonunions can be attributed to various causes—a naturally diminished blood supply to the area that existed even before the fracture, use of anti-inflammatory medications, nicotine use, poor immobilization, patients' failure to follow doctor's orders—or they can happen for no known reason. In such non-weight-bearing bones as the clavicle, a nonunion may cause no pain and allow the patient to continue to function normally. In such cases, no surgery is necessary. On the other hand, with fractures in a bone that bears weight, such as the femur, a nonunion must be surgically repaired to avoid dysfunction and pain. Rigid immobilization, through either insertion of a metal plate and screws or intramedullary nailing (insertion of a metal rod down the middle of the bone), is the treatment of choice.

Acute fractures rarely need any additional bone grafting techniques, whereas chronic fractures that have not healed will require it. Bone grafting can be done with an autograft (the patient's own bone), an allograft, (bone from a bone bank), bone paste, or synthetic bony material. In grafting nonunions, the surgeon removes the fibrous connection between the major fragments and as much unhealthy bone as possible without shortening

Bone Healing

the bone too much. The two ends are then set firmly together, by either plating or nailing. After which, the bone graft can be inserted. Most of the graft will be the softer inside (or cancellous, bone harvested from parts of the pelvis called the *iliac crests*). This bone is malleable and, after it is packed tightly around the prepared nonunion site, can be held in place by repaired periosteum. In the case of an autograft, the patient's own bone cells contained in the graft can promote healing, and in both an autograft and an allograft, the cancellous bone's consistency provides a framework to support new bone growth.

Does grafting always work? No. Nonunions can be the most difficult of all orthopaedic challenges. Despite the best techniques and the most rigid fixations and grafting, the bone may simply not heal. In some cases, the surgeon may attempt another procedure, but in my experience, the likelihood of failure rises with the number of attempts. Fortunately, unless a doctor specializes in trauma care, he or she will not see many nonunions in a normal practice.

CHAPTER 22
THE OPERATION

When someone is in need of orthopaedic surgery, appropriate preparations in the doctor's office should include the following:

- The doctor's describing to the patient the operation to be performed
- A discussion of potential complications and necessary rehabilitation
- Explanation and signing of appropriate consent forms
- Appropriate medical evaluations and tests prior to surgery
- Scheduling of the procedure with the hospital or surgical center
- Written preoperative and postoperative instructions for the patient

In the event of an *emergency* operation, these steps may have to be abbreviated and completed quickly. Most of this chapter has to do with *elective* surgery, meaning you and your doctor are choosing to arrange it at the convenience of both.

A word here about scheduling of the surgery is appropriate. Some cases may be scheduled as the hospital's first procedure of the day, requiring the patient to arrive at the hospital at what seems an ungodly hour of

The Operation

the morning. Other procedures are scheduled for later times based on an estimate of the first procedure's expected time of conclusion. I say *estimate* because a surgeon may normally take a certain time to perform a specific operation, but sometimes, there are glitches and unforeseen complications that add to the time needed to complete the procedure. If that happens, the following cases must be delayed. For that reason alone, it's always preferable to have your operation be the first one on the schedule, if it can be arranged. If yours is one of the later cases, you'll spend more time in the preoperative area, which can add to your anxiety.

Many hospitals ask someone awaiting surgery to come in several days ahead of time to take care of lab work and paperwork and check on insurance information. That relieves you of having to do it on the actual day of surgery, when you may be more anxious. Your doctor and the anesthesia service will want to know the results of your lab tests well in advance of the operation.

Information about your medical condition sent in by your medical doctor will be reviewed, and a representative of the hospital or surgery center will have you read and sign a consent form for the operation you're to undergo. I suggest you read this one very carefully and ask to have anything explained that you don't understand. Be sure the operation you discussed with your doctor is the same one specified on this form. If the operation is to be on an arm or a leg, be sure the correct side is specified. The possible complications your doctor discussed with you should be listed on the form. It should also include a statement saying you agree to allow the hospital to do certain things that your doctor may not have discussed with you.

If you have any questions, now is the time to ask them. If you need clarification from the hospital's point of view, ask the nurse who is assigned to your case. If you have questions concerning the operation, ask your doctor. At this time, a member of the anesthesiology service may visit you to explain what type of anesthesia will be used and find out whether you are allergic to particular drugs. You will also be told what precautions to take with eating or drinking on the night before the surgery and which of your medications you should or should not take that night or in the morning. Aspirin and blood-thinning medication (Coumadin, for example) can reduce your blood's ability to clot, so you will be cautioned about that.

On the day of surgery, after you check in, your doctor should come in and see you before you're given any medications so that you're coherent enough to understand any answers and fully capable of signing the consent form if you haven't done that already. You will have a bracelet on your wrist stating your name, date of birth, and doctor, and you should make sure the bracelet correctly identifies you. The nurse will also check it and ask you if it is correct. This bracelet will be on you for your entire stay in the hospital and usually will not be removed even when you leave. You or a family member can remove it once you're back at home.

Before you're given any medication, the nurse will ask you a lot of questions you may have already answered, including questions about your allergies and medications you're taking. She will want to ascertain whether you have recently taken any aspirin or blood thinner and whether you've had anything to eat or drink since midnight. This is very important. If you ate or drank anything after midnight other than a few sips of water, you could vomit during the procedure, drawing your stomach contents into your lungs. This *aspiration* is an utterly life-threatening condition. If you had anything to eat or drink after midnight, please be sure to notify both the nurse and your doctor. Depending on the type of surgery and the anesthesia planned, your operation may have to be canceled for your own protection. It's not worth taking your life in your hands by misinforming the nurse about this issue.

While some patients are under the impression that they are having minor surgery or major surgery, I was never comfortable with this wording. I suppose an operation with local anesthesia could be considered minor, as the patient is awake, the surgery may not be a lengthy one, and the patient may expect to go home on the day of surgery. Any surgery can have complications, however, as all surgeons know. Patients should be aware of it too. Once a complication occurs, that surgery suddenly becomes major in my mind. For that reason, in my practice, all surgeries were major to me and my patients.

If you're to have an arm or leg operated on, the nurse may give you a marking pen and have you write "yes" on the correct extremity and "no" on the opposite one to avoid a mistake in the operating room. Once all these matters have been attended to, the nurse will start an intravenous (meaning "in the vein," an IV) access that is connected to a mixture of saline or glucose water. Usually, the IV needle, with its plastic sheath, will be inserted into the arm. Once the needle is in a vein, it can be removed, leaving in place a more flexible plastic tube. The nurse will tape the IV in place to make sure it isn't pulled out by accident. After that, you'll receive medications necessary for your operation, such as antibiotics and anesthetics, through this IV.

If your preoperative blood studies reveal any values below normal—a low red-blood cell count, for example—repeat studies may be ordered to check your present values. No anesthetic or mind-altering medications will be given until you have seen your doctor and had all your questions and concerns answered.

If you didn't see a member of the anesthesia service at your earlier preoperative visit to the hospital, an anesthesiologist or certified registered nurse anesthetist will visit you and probably ask you some of the same questions you've already answered. It may seem time wasted, but it's important because you, in your nervous state, might forget to mention an allergy or condition to one person and remember it later. They will ask about previous surgeries and whether you had any problems with the anesthesia used. They will want you to open your mouth wide to see if your mouth and throat will admit an adequate airway. And then you wait.

When it's time for you to be rolled to the operating room, you may be given a relaxing medication through your IV. The anesthesiologist and a nurse will usually accompany you. Your doctor may walk along with you as well, unless he or she is scrubbing—thoroughly cleansing hands and arms—in preparation for your surgery. In the operating room, you will be transferred to an operating table that may be narrower than you expected. You will be helped to center yourself on this table, and then your arms will be spread outward.

If you're to undergo local anesthesia, a nurse may be with you but no anesthetist. If you're to have general anesthesia, however, the anesthetist will be at your head guiding you through each maneuver performed, such as the attachment of a blood pressure cuff, a heart monitor, or a temperature gauge. Once everything is fully prepared, the anesthetist will tell you that you're about to be given medication through your IV that will put you to sleep. A mask will be placed over your nose and mouth, loose enough to allow you to get plenty of oxygen into your lungs. You will probably not remember anything that happens after these last few minutes.

Once you are fully anesthetized, normally, a plastic *endotracheal* [en-doh-TRAY-kee-al] tube will be passed through your mouth into your windpipe, or *trachea* [TRAY-kee-ah], past your vocal cords, and into the large conduit of the lungs, the *mainstem bronchus* [BRON-kuss]. A small balloon on the end will be inflated to hold the endotracheal tube in place, and tape will be placed on this tube outside your mouth for the same reason. Some moisturizing paste will be placed in your eyes, and they will be taped shut.

If it is necessary to position your body specifically for your operation, you will be moved into the position your surgeon requires. Most of the time, the surgeon or his team will supervise this maneuvering. Any areas of abnormal pressure will be cushioned and protected. Once all this is completed, the operative area of your arm, leg, neck, or back will be *prepped*—that is, washed with antiseptic soap or liquid, possibly followed by alcohol. Any area near the operative site not to be included in the operation will be draped off and covered with a sterile towel or sheet, leaving only the operative site visible. This area may then be covered with a sterile transparent plastic material that adheres to your skin. The operative site is now ready.

These preparations take quite a long time. Everyone has his job in the operating room. Everything must be checked and double-checked. If there is an accidental break in sterility—if some previous sterile surface has been contaminated—it must all be done over from the beginning, and that can take a long time. That's one reason that a 7:30 a.m. operation that's supposed to last an hour may not end at 8:30 a.m. The stated time of one hour was probably the surgical time, not counting all the preoperative preparation. The skin incision for a surgery scheduled at 7:30 a.m. may not begin for half an hour to forty-five minutes after the start time.

Should a spinal anesthetic be needed, that takes more time too. You will be asked to lie on your side with your knees drawn toward your chest so your back can be prepped. Some spinals are administered while you are sitting and hunched over. Drapes will be applied. The anesthesiologist will apply a numbing medicine to your skin and then place a spinal needle between the spinous processes of your middle lower back. The needle will not injure the spinal cord itself, as the actual spinal cord will be well above the area of needle entrance.

The outside covering of the spinal cord is called the *dura* [DOO-rah], so the space outside the dura is called the *epidural* space. After the spinal needle enters this space, a catheter is passed through the needle into the space, the needle is removed, and the anesthetic medication is injected. The catheter is taped to your back with an attached syringe containing more of the anesthetic medication if needed. A period of time will elapse before the medication begins to do its job. Once it takes effect, your legs will be numb and paralyzed until the operation is over and for several hours thereafter.

A variety of local anesthetic techniques known as *regional anesthetic blocks* are used in the upper extremities, some of the common ones being supraclavicular, axillary, and Bier blocks. These are administered by an anesthesiologist. Supraclavicular and axillary blocks are carried out by placing a needle either above the clavicle for the *supraclavicular* block or in the armpit for the *axillary* block. A Bier block is an intravenous anesthetic technique under tourniquet control, usually in the arm. A needle is placed in the back of the hand or in the forearm near the hand. A wrap is then applied around the arm, beginning at the hand and ending at the middle upper arm, in an attempt to push all the blood out of the veins of the arm and back into the body. With the wrapping intact, a tourniquet is inflated to keep any blood from flowing back into the arm. The wrapping is then removed and a local anesthetic medication is injected into the empty veins of the arm to numb the arm from the elbow down. This technique is used for operations that will last no more than an hour and a half. After the operation, the tourniquet is released and blood flows into the arm, washing out the anesthetic so that normal feeling soon returns.

Now for a discussion of how surgical wounds are closed. You'll recall our discussion of arthroscopic procedures in which the surgeon inserts a scope into a joint to inspect the joint's interior. These procedures are carried out through small incisions, possibly more than two depending on the operation. The surgeon usually closes the incisions with a suture and applies a compression dressing.

Open surgeries are those that require a skin incision of some length. For some open surgeries, the surgeon will close the tissue under the skin with an absorbable suture and close the skin incision with metal staples or non-absorbable sutures. For most of my open surgeries, I used metal staples, both for ease of application and for a smoother, more cosmetically pleasing result. Some physicians close the skin with a *subcuticular* [sub-kew-TICK-yew-lar] stitch, a continuous suture that stitches the more superficial layer of subcutaneous tissue and is visible only at each end of the wound. Other shorter incisions may be closed subcutaneously with several sutures and *Steri-strips*, small strips of white tape over the skin. The surgeon may also wish to immobilize your operated arm or leg.

With the operation complete, your anesthesiologist will begin waking you in the operating room. He waits to remove the endotracheal tube until it is obvious that you are awake enough to breathe on your own, all the while monitoring your vital signs (heart rate, blood pressure, blood oxygen level) and reactions to waking up.

You are then transferred to a rolling stretcher and taken to the recovery room or postoperative area. Another nurse is assigned to your case and watches you carefully for anything out of the ordinary, and your vital signs are continuously monitored. As you gradually become lucid, you'll be asked how you're feeling, if you have pain, if you can feel your fingers or toes, if you can move parts of your body that are not close to the area that was operated on.

Once you're awake, your doctor may talk to you, but if not, he will have talked to your family members and told them how the surgery progressed and how you fared throughout it. As you recuperate, your doctor may already be performing another procedure and may even still be operating when you're ready to go home or have returned to your hospital room. This is the reason she or he may not speak with you after the operation, but definite instructions will have been left with regard to your care, which you'll be told about. An office appointment time may have already been made for you, or you may need to schedule your own appointment to visit the doctor soon after your surgery.

Your IV will be removed only when the hospital personnel believe everything to be satisfactory. You will then be allowed to sit up. Don't expect to stand or walk immediately. Just sitting up may make some patients dizzy or even nauseated. This may occur several times until you can sit up without feeling unwell. At that point, you may need to visit the bathroom and should insist on having a nurse go with you. The nurse will decide whether you can walk or need a wheelchair to get there.

Finally, you will be able to go. You'll be given final instructions on caring for your operative site and probably a prescription for pain medication.

Normally, a member of the hospital or surgery center staff will wheel you to the car in which a family member or friend will drive you home. If your knee, ankle, or foot was operated on, as soon as you reach home, you should elevate the leg to keep down swelling and keep it elevated as much as possible.

No matter what procedure you had, you should check your bandage for bleeding. Occasionally after an operation, a small vessel may start to bleed and you may see blood inside or on your bandage. If that happens, notify your doctor or go to his office and ask to see him or a member of his staff so that the bandage can be checked. If this happens at night, you may be better off going to the emergency room to be evaluated.

If you're concerned, don't hesitate to have someone check your wound. That's always the safe thing to do. Better safe than sorry is the rule. My employees, partners, and I were all on the same page when it came to any potential postoperative complications. Any of our patients who reported such concerns were told to come into the office for an evaluation immediately. We almost always had a surgeon there, so I believe our patients were evaluated and treated appropriately. I can't remember a time in my thirty years in practice that a postoperative patient of mine who complained of something out of the ordinary was not promptly evaluated by someone in our practice.

The Operation

One more word about the consent form. Some physicians, after describing the procedure and its risks and benefits, have you sign their consent form in addition to the consent form you sign for the hospital or surgery center. I took it a bit further.

When I anticipated an operation on a shoulder—my subspecialty—an ACL reconstruction, or a total joint replacement, I would set up a meeting for patients with the same disorder after office hours when I had plenty of time for discussion. As I had many rotator cuff and other common shoulder procedures to discuss with a good many patients, I would invite as many as five patients and a family member each, if possible, to a roundtable discussion where I would review the anatomy of the affected joint with diagrams and models, discuss their specific problems, explain how I would go about evaluating and treating their malady, discuss how much pain they might expect, tell them what else to expect postoperatively, and describe at length the necessary rehabilitation. At the end of the conference, after answering all their questions, I handed them a list of the subjects discussed and asked them to sign the form. Some large hospitals have similar preoperative classes.

Most patients enjoyed knowing more about their problem than just the diagnosis and surgery involved. They enjoyed their interaction with others who were experiencing similar problems, pain, and lifestyle disturbance. They went away from these discussions less anxious and less fearful, and I believe I taught them something more than they would have learned elsewhere. Most physicians don't have such discussions. I just had the time and the proper patient population to do so. It worked very well for my patients and me. They had their questions answered, and my discussions with them were all well documented.

CHAPTER 23
STUDIES AND TESTS

Orthpaedists, like general practitioners and other specialists, use various studies and techniques to diagnose patients' complaints. Those commonly employed in the field of orthopaedic surgery are listed here:

History

I consider obtaining a careful patient history, along with a thorough physical examination, the most important technique of all. Unfortunately, the advent of a wealth of technological advancements in my specialty may have led some physicians to drift away from the gold standard of a comprehensive history and physical examination.

One of my medical school professors told his students, "Listen to the patient; he's telling you the diagnosis." He was absolutely correct. At that time, however, I didn't realize that every condition and complaint could be surrounded by a maze that we physicians must work our way through by asking appropriate questions to reach the heart of the maze: the diagnosis. Asking the right questions helps to smooth the effort for both patient and doctor, while asking the wrong questions or no questions at all may not yield a true diagnosis. The art of taking a good history isn't taught in medical school. It comes through practice, understanding what you did right and especially what you did wrong, and evaluating a myriad of disease processes many times over. Maybe this is the reason we use the word *practice* to describe what we do!

Some patients have no idea how to voice their complaints. For instance, my father-in-law was one of the smartest men I've ever known, but I found getting him to actually answer a question about his symptoms to be almost impossible. He didn't use the word *pain* but rather referred to "an uncomfortable feeling," "a pressure," "an ache," or "something weird going on" in his body. When asked about pain, he would say he had none. Asking him the appropriate questions was quite a challenge, as it is with many people. We physicians tend to categorize our thinking as well as questioning and expect the patient's answer to fit our expectations, but if the patient's answers don't fit our categories or our terminology, we may take far too long to get to the diagnosis or never arrive at it at all.

Physical Examination

A comprehensive examination *with repetition* is essential. I emphasize repetition because repeating certain portions of the exam, if not all, allows the doctor to confirm his findings. All normal findings should be reexamined to be sure they are normal. This sounds like a waste of time, but it is extremely important.

For example, the "white coat syndrome," heightened anxiety at being in the doctor's office, can cause the patient to voluntarily tense his or her muscles in a way that makes a particular joint seem to be normal, but if the patient can be persuaded to relax later in the exam, evidence of instability in that joint may emerge. An examination of the area just above the affected joint may help rule out a referred pain pattern. Such an exam could allow for a comparison of motion of the joint in question with the opposite side.

The ability to put a patient who is in pain at ease is truly an art. Most of the time, I thought I had this ability, but with some patients, it was never easy; with others, never achievable. There were plenty of times, however, when I could help the patient relax sufficiently to reveal physical findings important to the diagnosis. There were many times when patients who saw me for second opinions told me the physicians who had examined them initially had not been as thorough as I was. I say this not to boast but to support my belief that other physicians may not have considered a thorough physical examination as important as I did.

Arthrocentesis

Arthrocentesis [R-throw-sen-tee-sis] means using a needle and syringe to aspirate fluid from a joint. Aspiration in an orthopaedic practice refers to removal of fluid from a joint or a space as well. We use this technique to relieve fluid buildup inside a joint, remove blood from joints, remove blood from hematomas, and obtain fluid for microscopic evaluation. If infection is suspected, the fluid can be cultured to tell us if a bacterial process is present, what organism it is, and to what antibiotic it is sensitive. If we suspect gout, microscopic examination may reveal uric acid crystals, and if we suspect another disease such as pseudo-gout, the exam may show calcium pyrophosphate crystals. The same needling technique is used to inject fluid, such as a refined steroid, an antibiotic, or a visco-supplement, into a joint.

X-ray Studies

As most folks who have seen an orthopaedic physician know, radiologic or X-ray examination is an orthopaedist's bread-and-butter technique. Most orthopaedists today have the necessary equipment and personnel to carry out radiologic examinations in the office. These are taken with the special film inside a cassette, under or behind the part to be X-rayed, and the film is retrieved in a dark room and placed in a developer. The film is then dropped outside the dark room sixty to ninety seconds later for review by the physician. Today, digital radiography, the X-ray image appears on a screen for the physician's review with no actual film. The great advantage of this method is that the image can be sent elsewhere electronically for a second opinion if necessary while the patient is still in the office. Some hospitals have this ability and are also able to give the patient a CD with a copy of the completed X-ray study, which the physician can examine on his own computer.

To make a useful X-ray study, the technician positions the patient with the affected bone or joint in various positions for the fullest evaluation of the problem. An X-ray study in one position may be *negative* (normal) while some other position might yield a *positive* (or abnormal) view. Thus for the most complete evaluation, more than one X-ray may be required in more than one position.

Arthrography

This specialized X-ray study makes use of a fluid that is *radio-opaque*— that is, it obstructs the passage of the X-ray beam. When injected into a joint, this fluid, which appears bright white on the X-ray image, can reveal structures within the joint that are not otherwise visible. Before newer techniques were invented, these *arthrogram* studies of the shoulder and the knee were done routinely. For many years, I used the technique almost exclusively with shoulder problems, devising my own variant of it by adding lidocaine to give me more information than either an MRI or a CAT scan could. Because lidocaine is a local anesthetic, by numbing the joint during the X-ray evaluation, I was able to determine whether the patient's pain emanated from the joint itself or had some other origin. Today, however, arthrography is not performed very much as the more technical MRI and CAT scan have taken its place.

Bone Scan

A bone scan is used to distinguish among areas of normal, increased, and decreased bone metabolism. It is generally used to identify abnormal processes involving the bone, such as tumor and tumor spread, infection, and fracture. To carry out the study, a *radiotracer*, a radioactive solution absorbed by bone, must be injected into a vein. A camera then slowly scans the body, taking pictures that indicate the amount of radiotracer absorbed by various areas of bone. Orthopaedists use this study mostly for stress fractures, tumors, avascular necrosis, and unidentified bone pain. A technique known as a three-phase bone scan is used to look for bone infections. The images are taken shortly after injection of the radioactive material.

Computerized Axial Tomography (CAT scan or CT scan)

This technique is the next step up from the general X-ray study, which uses a stationary X-ray machine to focus beams of radiation on a particular area of the body, producing one-dimensional images on X-ray film. The CAT machine has a computer unit inside and a X-ray unit that rotates around the body so that it produces a set of cross-sectional images of the scanned area that can be thought of as pictorial slices of the inside of your body. Orthopaedists use CAT scans mostly for complicated fractures, dislocations, and tumors.

Magnetic Resonance Imagery (MRI)

Magnetic Resonance Imagery, which provides detailed images of the body in any plane, is most commonly used to investigate the body's structure and function. An MRI study provides a much greater contrast between the different soft tissues of the body than the CAT scan, making it especially useful in studying the brain and soft tissues such as tendon and ligaments and menisci, in cardiovascular applications, and in cancer patients. Unlike the CAT scan, it uses no ionizing radiation—that is, no X-rays are emitted. Instead, the machine creates a magnetic field that aligns nuclear magnetized hydrogen atoms in the water in the body. Too technical to explain, but suffice it to say that orthopaedists use MRI studies to evaluate spine conditions, herniated discs, cartilage tears in the knee, rotator cuff and labral tears in the shoulder, and other disorders in all bones and joints.

Positron Emission Tomography (PET scan)

A PET scan is a unique imaging test that helps doctors see how the organs and tissues in your body are actually functioning. It has nothing to do with your pet although the first free-standing PET-scan facility in my town *was* right next door to an animal hospital. For years, patients would ask me what kind of imaging device those veterinarians were using.

Like with a bone scan, a radioactive chemical called a tracer is injected into a patient's vein, traveling through the body to be absorbed by the organs and tissues under study. The scanner machine detects and records the energy given off by the tracer substance and converts it into three-dimensional pictures. A physician can then look at cross-sectional images of the body organ from any angle to detect any functional problems.

While a PET scan can measure blood flow, oxygen use, and glucose metabolism, helping doctors distinguish between normally and abnormally functioning organs and tissues, at this writing, it has very little to offer the orthopaedist. I imagine that a modification of this scan technology may pop up in the near future that will give us an even greater ability to picture our patients' bones and joints without having to perform invasive tests.

Venous Doppler Examination and Ultrasonography.

For a venous Doppler test, high-frequency sound waves applied to parts of the body yield pictures of the inside of the body.

Ultrasound examinations, unlike X-ray studies, do not use ionizing radiation, or are they an invasive type of test. As ultrasound images show what is happening in real time, they reveal the structure and movement of the body's internal organs as well as the flow of blood through blood vessels. The two methods may be combined as with a Doppler ultrasound study to evaluate blood as it flows through a blood vessel. Orthopaedists use this technology mostly to evaluate deep vein *thromboses* or blood clots within the calf. Some have developed ultrasound for the rotator cuff and other areas as well.

Arthroscopy

Early in the 1970s, arthroscopy was a diagnostic technique used exclusively for the knee. Insertion of the arthroscope through very small incisions allowed the surgeon to perform a diagnostic examination of the knee to determine what was wrong, providing better visualization of the joint than an open surgical procedure could.

Ultimately, better instrumentation and smaller video cameras and monitors allowed us to use the arthroscope to evaluate many joints in the body and perform operations similar to their open counterparts but with less tissue destruction. Newer surgical procedures quickly evolved that, in the 1970s, would never have been thought possible but are now routine. This improved technology has made it possible to uncover previously unknown disease processes and diagnose soft-tissue damage, giving us a better understanding of the miracles of joints and other spaces in the body. Fiber optic technology is now being used by almost every other specialty.

While some open procedures are still necessary, such arthroscopically assisted procedures as ACL reconstruction and mini-open procedures of the shoulder often produce better results than the open procedures of the past. There are, however, some drawbacks. Of the newer crop of orthopaedic surgeons, almost all are trained in programs that make primary use of arthroscopy. Open procedures, especially those for the shoulder, are being performed less often, and the new generations of surgeons may eventually not know how to perform them. In years to come, if an arthroscopic repair fails, an open procedure may be required, but who will know the ins and outs and have the necessary depth of experience to perform them? This is my concern for the future of orthopaedic surgery.

AFTERWORD

I hope your knowledge of orthopaedic conditions of the body has been enhanced. After all, that was the sole intention of this book. With the knowledge you now have, you should be able to communicate more effectively with your physician and understand more about your problem. I see no reason why this knowledge will not increase your chances of obtaining a quicker and definitive diagnosis of your condition.

Thank you for taking the time to read this guide.

GLOSSARY

Abduction: Positioning part of the body away from the midline of the body or from a neighboring part or limb of the body

Acute tendinitis: Inflammation of a tendon or its lining with a sudden onset

Acromio-clavicular arthroplasty: An operation on the acromio-clavicular (A-C) joint

Acromio-clavicular (A-C) joint: The joint at the distal end, or outside edge, of the clavicle

Acromion process: The bony process of the scapula over the shoulder that forms the outside of the A-C joint

Acromioplasty: An operation to remove and flatten the undersurface of the acromion

Adduction: Positioning part of the body toward the midline of the body or from a neighboring part or limb of the body

Adhesive capsulitis: A stiff and painful self-limiting disease of the shoulder

Adipose tissue: Fatty tissue

ALPSA (Anterior Labro-ligamentous Periosteal Sleeve Avulsion) lesion: A defect caused by an anterior dislocation, or subluxation, of the shoulder

Angina pectoris: Chest pain caused by heart disease

Annulus fibrosis: Fibrous material surrounding the center of a vertebral disc

Anterior: Any area located in front of the body as it is positioned with the palms and forearms facing forward

Anterior dislocation: A complete separation of a joint with the distal, or farther, part located toward the front of the body

Arthrodesis: A surgical procedure to fuse bones together

Arthrography/Arthrogram: A radiologic study performed by injecting contrast within a joint

Arthroplasty: A surgical procedure on a joint

Arthroscopy: A surgical procedure for visualizing and operating on the inside of a joint using fibro-optic instrumentation, a light source, and a viewing monitor

Articular cartilage: A hyaline cartilage covering of the end of any bone forming a joint

Aseptic necrosis: A noninfectious bone-death process

Atrophy: A wasting away of a part of the body, especially muscle

Avascular necrosis: A noninfectious bone death process

Bankart lesion: A defect in the humeral head caused by an anterior dislocation, or subluxation, of the shoulder

Biceps muscle: The muscle in the anterior aspect of the upper arm with two muscle bellies

Bicipital groove: The groove through which the long head of the biceps tendon exits the shoulder joint

Bursa: A two-layered sac found in many areas of the body that helps tissues to glide on one another with a minimum of friction

Bursitis: Inflammation of a bursa

Capitellum: The lateral aspect of the end of the humerus forming part of the elbow joint

Carpal tunnel syndrome: Compression of the median nerve in the carpal canal of the wrist

Cauterization: The act of using a controlled electric current in surgery to stop bleeding

Chronic tendinitis: A long-term presence of an inflammatory process of a tendon

Chondromalacia: Fragmentation of articular (hyaline) cartilage

Clavicle: The collarbone

Complete rotator cuff tear (RCT): A full thickness defect of any rotator cuff tendon

Contusion: A superficial small collection of blood under the skin and in the fatty tissue beneath

Coraco-acromial ligament: The ligament connecting the undersurface of the clavicle to the coracoid process of the scapula

Coracoid process: An anterior bony projection of the scapula; the short head of the biceps muscle origination site

Core decompression: A surgical procedure to drill out the center of a bone, usually the femoral head, in an attempt to stimulate a blood supply

Cortical bone: The hard outside portion of bone

Crepitus: Crunching, either heard or felt, from inside or outside a body part

Cubital tunnel: The tunnel the ulnar nerve occupies on the posterior medial side of the elbow

Cyst: A fluid-filled sac

Degenerative disc: The end result of the fragmentation of an intervertebral disc

Degenerative spondylolithesis: The sliding forward of one vertebra on another caused by degenerative changes in the spine, usually in the lower back

Deltoideus or deltoid muscle: The large muscle on the outside of the upper arm that lifts the arm from the body's side

Desiccation: The act of drying

Dermatomal pattern: The specific areas of skin supplied by different nerves

Dislocation: The complete separation of one part of a joint from another

Distal: The most distant part of a bone or body part

Distal interpahalangeal joint: The joint at the end of each finger or toe

Dorsal: Posterior, when used in describing the upper extremity

Dorsiflexion: Backward bending of a joint such as the wrist; upward motion of the ankle

Ecchymosis: The presence of black and blue discoloration

Etiology: The causation of a disease

Extensor carpi radialis brevis: One of the muscles that dorsiflexes the wrist

Extensor tendon: A tendon connected to any muscle that extends or straightens a joint

External rotation: The active or passive motion causing an extremity to rotate away from the midline of that part

External rotation by the side: The act of external rotation while the arm is by the side of the body

Extra-articular: Immediately outside a joint

Femoral condyles: The two projections at the distal end of the femur forming the upper part of the knee joint

Femoral head: The ball-like top of the femur bone forming part of the hip

Femoral neck: The portion of bone between the femoral head and the rest of the femur

Femur: The thigh bone

Fibocartilage: Cartilage formed mostly by fibrous material

Fibrosis: Scarring

Flexion contracture: The loss of a joint's ability to fully extend, secondary to tightness of the ligaments or bony deformity

Fluoroscopy: A radiologic technique whereby real-time motion can be visualized

Frozen shoulder: A term used for any condition causing loss of motion of the shoulder, Adhesive Capsulitis

Glenoid: The lateral socket formation of the scapula forming part of the ball and socket formation of the shoulder joint

Glenoid labrum: A circumferential rim of fibrocartilage around the glenoid cavity of the shoulder and hip socket

Gluteus medius: A muscle in the hip area that abducts the femur

Greater occipital nerve: A cranial nerve that supplies sensation to the back of the skull

Greater tuberosity: The lateral portion of the humeral head onto which three rotator-cuff tendons insert

Guyon's canal: A wrist tunnel through which the ulnar nerve traverses to enter the hand

Hematoma: A collection of blood

Herniated disc: The partial or complete displacement of a disc from its original position within the intervertebral space

Hill-Sachs lesion: A notch defect in the posterior aspect of the humeral head caused by compression by the anterior glenoid with an anterior dislocation of the shoulder

Humeral head: The hemispherical shape at the very top of the upper arm bone (the humerus) forming part of the shoulder joint

Humerus: The upper arm bone

Hyaline cartilage: The smooth, white, glistening coverage on the ends of all bones that form a joint

Idiopathic: Having no specific cause

Ilio-tibial band of the fascia lata: The long flat tendon on the lateral (outside) part of the hip and thigh inserting on the outside of the tibia just below the knee

Impingement syndrome: A condition of the shoulder causing irritation of the rotator cuff by a compression phenomenon between the acromion and the humeral head.

Incomplete tear of the rotator cuff (IRCT): A partial defect (less than full thickness) of the rotator cuff

Inferior: The bottom or at the bottom of any structure; the opposite of *superior*

Infraspinatus: One of the rotator cuff muscles

Internal rotation: The active or passive act of rotating an extremity toward the midline of the body

Intervertebral disc: The structure formed by nucleus pulposus and annulus fibrosis

Intra-articular: Inside a joint

Intra-tendinous: Inside a tendon

Glossary

Ischial tuberosity: A bony process found on the inferior aspect of the pelvis where the hamstring tendons originate

Joint capsule: The ligamentous structures completely surrounding a joint

Labro-ligamentous complex: A structure formed by ligaments originating from a labrum

Lateral: The portion of a body part farther out from the midline

Lateral epicondylitis: Tennis elbow

Lateral cutaneous nerve: The nerve that supplies the sensation to the anterior lateral aspect of the thigh

Lateral malleolus: The distal end of the fibula forming the lateral wall of the ankle joint

Lateral recess: The tunnel area through which spinal nerves traverse as they exit the spinal canal

Lesser trochanter: The posterior medial bony projection just below the femoral neck upon to which the iliopsoas muscle inserts

Lesser tuberosity: The anterior aspect of the humeral head upon to which the subscapularis tendon inserts

Lidocaine: A short-acting local-anesthetic injectable fluid

Ligamentum flavum: The ligament between the posterior arches of each vertebra

Loculated: Having multiple small spaces walled off from one another in a larger area such as a cyst or a tumor

Longitudinal ligament: The posterior ligament connecting the vertebrae of the spine

Long head of the biceps: The lateral muscle belly of the biceps muscle whose tendon originates in the shoulder joint

Lunate bone: One of the carpal bones of the wrist

Mallet finger: Deformity of the tip of the finger as a result of an extensor tendon rupture

Marcaine: A long-acting local anesthetic injectable fluid

Massive tear: A rotator cuff defect greater than 5 centimeters in any direction

Medial: The part of an extremity closest to the midline of the body

Medial malleolus: The medial projection of the distal end of the tibia forming the medial wall of the ankle joint

Medial epicondyle: The bony prominence of the inner aspect of the humerus at the elbow

Median nerve: The nerve supplying the sensation to the volar aspect of the thumb, the index and middle fingers, and the lateral aspect of the ring finger

Medullary bone: The portion of bone inside the cortical (hard) bone

Metacarpal: Pertaining to the long bones of the hand
Metacarpo-phalangeal joint: The large joints of the hand, knuckles
Metatarsal : Pertaining to the bones of the foot
Metatarso-phalangeal joint: Pertaining to the joints between the foot and toes
Negative pressure: The pressure within a joint such as the hip that gives the joint stability beyond its ligamentous structures
Neurologic deficit: Any objective weakness, loss of sensation, loss of position sense, or loss of tendon reflex caused by a nerve dysfunction
Neuropathy: Any noninfectious disease of nerve
Nucleus pulposus: The elastic semifluid mass in the center of an intervertebral disc
Objective: physically identifiable
Olecranon bursitis: Inflammation of the bursa over the olecranon process of the elbow
Olecranon process of the ulna: The proximal tip of the ulna at the elbow
Ossify: To form bone
Osteonecrosis: The death of bone
Palpate: Physical examination using the hands
Panner's disease: A juvenile self-limiting disease of the capitellum of the elbow
Pars intraarticularis: The portion of the vertebral arch nearest the vertebra
Paravertebral: Area next to the vertebral spine
Plantar-flexion: The downward motion of the ankle
Plasma: That part of blood without blood cells
Posterior: Positioned behind or toward the back of a part; the opposite of anterior
Posterior dislocation: Dislocation involving the distal part of a joint being fully separated from its joint posteriorly
Prone: Lying on one's stomach; the opposite of *supine*
Proximal: That part of a bone closest to the body along the bones axis
Proximal interphalangeal joint: The finger joint just distal to the knuckle
Radial deviation: Tilting of the hand to the radial or medial side of the wrist
Radio-opaque: Able to absorb radiation
Radius: The bone of the forearm that rotates about the ulna
Recurrent subluxations or dislocations: Subluxations/dislocations that occur more than once
Referred pain: Pain located in any area not near the actual physical source of the pain

Rib hump: The enlarged exaggeration of the rib cage on one side as a result of scoliosis

Rotator cuff: Four tendons connected to muscles that affect the multiple motions of the shoulder

Rotator-cuff tear: Degenerative fragmentation of a rotator cuff tendon

Scaphoid bone: One of the carpal bones of the wrist, also known as the navicular

Scapho-lunate ligament: The ligament connecting the scaphoid and lunate bones of the wrist

Scapula: The shoulder blade

Spinal stenosis: A degenerative condition of the spine causing compression of nerves and tissues

Spinous process: The most posterior aspect of the vertebral arch

Spondylolisthesis: The result of one vertebra's sliding forward or backward on the vertebra below

Spondylolysis: A developmental defect or crack of the pars interarticularis

Stenosing tenosynovitis: Tendon inflammation in a confined space

Stenosis: Narrowing of a tunnel, canal, or outlet

Subacromial bursa: The bursa present under the acromion and over the rotator cuff

Subluxation: Partial dislocation of a joint

Subscapularis: The most anterior of the rotator-cuff muscles originating from the anterior aspect of the scapula

Subcutaneous: Under the skin

Subjective: Felt by the patient but not necessarily identifiable on physical examination

Superior: The top or at the top of any structure; the opposite of *inferior*

Supraspinatus: The most superior of the rotator-cuff muscles

Supinate: To rotate the palm upward

Supine: Lying on one's back; the opposite of *prone*

Symphysis pubis: The anterior connection of the two pelvic wings

Synovium: The lining of a joint

Synovial fluid: The fluid manufactured by the synovium that nourishes the hyaline cartilage and menisci of joints

Synovial sheath: The lining of a tendon or tendon sheath

Talus: One of three bones forming the ankle joint

Tamponade effect: The cessation of bleeding caused by the pressure built up by blood in a confined space

Tenodesis: Attaching a tendon to bone or soft tissue

Tenolysis: Surgical removal of the lining of a tendon

Tendon reflex: The reactionary effect obtained by tapping on a tendon, such as a knee jerk elicited by striking the kneecap tendon

Tendinosis: Thickened degenerative tendon

Teres minor: A rotator cuff muscle, one of four

Thorax: The entire rib cage and thoracic spine

Thoracic spine: The twelve vertebra with rib connections

Tibia: The shinbone

Tibial plateau: The top of the tibia, on which the femoral condyles rest, forming the knee

Transverse carpal ligament: The ligament covering the carpal canal, through which traverse the median nerve and tendons to the fingers

Trapezius: The large muscle at the base of the neck projecting over to the shoulder

Trapezii: The plural of trapezius

Trapezium: A carpal bone of the wrist; also known as the greater multangular bone

Trigger point: A tender, painful area related to a specific process

Trigger finger: The snapping sensation in a finger as it is extended

Ulnar deviation: The lateral tilting (toward the ulna) of the hand at the wrist

Ulnar nerve: The "funny bone" nerve at the elbow that eventually traverses into the hand

Ulnar nerve subluxation: The partial dislocation of the ulnar nerve from its canal at the elbow

Volar: Anterior when describing the upper extremity

Volar flexion: The downward bending of the hand at the wrist

BIBLIOGRAPHY

1. Codman, E. A. *The Shoulder*, 1934, pg. 98, Thomas Todd Co., Printers, Boston MA.
2. Neviaser, J.S. *Arthrography of the Shoulder, the diagnosis and management of the lesions visualized,* 1962, Charles Thomas Publisher
3. Neviaser, T.J., Neviaser, R.J, Neviaser, J.S. - *Incomplete Rotator Cuff Tears: Technique for diagnosis and treatment,* Clinical Orthopedics & Related Research, 1994 Sept. (306) 12-16
4. Murthi AM, Vosburgh CL & Neviaser TJ. The incidence of pathologic changes of long head of the biceps tendon. J Shoulder Elbow Surg, 2000,9: 382-385.
5. Neviaser, T.J, Neviaser, R.J., Neviaser, J.S. *The Four-In-One Arthroplasty for the Painful Arc Syndrome,* Clinical Orthopedics & Related Research, 1982 Mar; (163):107-12
6. Perthes, G.C. Uber Operationen bei Habitueller Schulterluxation; Deutsche Zeitschrift fur Chirurgie, Leipzig, 1906, 85:199-227
7. Bankart, A.S.B. Recurrent Habitual Dislocation of the Shoulder. *British Medical Journal* 11, 1132, 1923
8. Neviaser, T. J. The Anterior Labro-Ligamentous Periosteal Sleeve Avulsion, A Case of Anterior Instability of the Shoulder: Arthroscopy 9: 17-21, 1993
9. Neviaser, T.J. The G.L.A.D. Lesion, Another Cause of Anterior Shoulder Pain: Arthroscopy 9, pg. 22, 1993
10. Neviaser, T.J. Adhesive Capsulitis: Operative Arthroscopy, Edition 2, New York, Raven Press; 1996, 785-91
11. Neviaser, J.S. Adhesive Capsulitis of the Shoulder. A Study of the Pathological Findings in Periarthritis of the Shoulder, J. Bone Joint Surgery, 27:211-222; 1945
12. Neviaser, T.J. Lateral Epicondylitis: Results of Outpatient Surgery and Immediate Motion; Contemporary Orthopedics 1985; 11:43–46